THE VAGUS NERVE

THE VAGUS NERVE

Unleashing the Body's Secret Weapon Against Disease

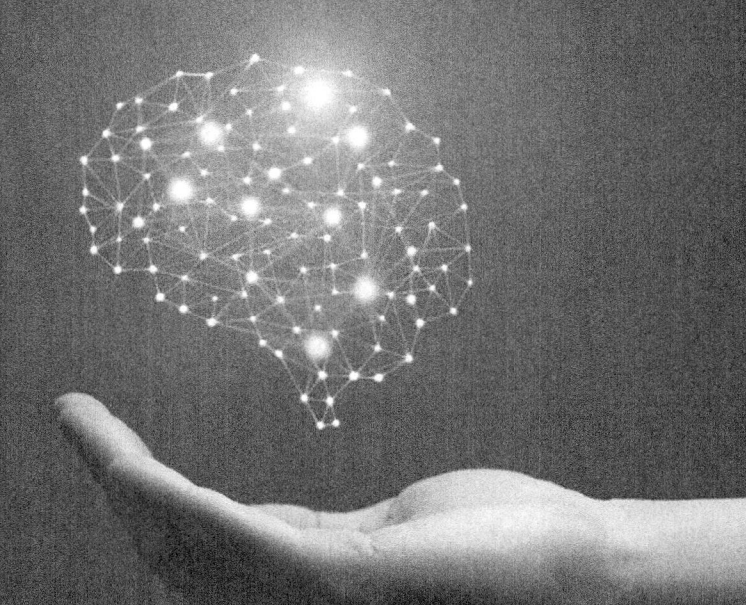

EMRYS GOLDSWORTHY

THE VAGUS NERVE

Unleashing the Body's Secret

Weapon Against Disease

EMRYS GOLDSWORTHY

Disclaimer

This book, including its content, information, advice, and recommendations, is intended to be used solely as a general educational aid and not for the purpose of providing medical or professional advice or services. The information provided in this book is not a substitute for professional care, and you should not use the information in place of a visit, consultation, diagnosis, or the advice of your physician or other healthcare providers.

The author and publisher of this book are not licensed medical professionals and make no representations or warranties of any kind in relation to this book and its contents and disclaim all responsibility and liability, including negligence, medical, or any other, arising in connection with the use of or reliance on any information, advice, or recommendations in this book. The author and publisher do not endorse or recommend any specific tests, products, procedures, opinions, or other information mentioned herein.

Readers should always seek the advice of their physician or qualified health provider with any questions they may have regarding a medical condition or treatment and before undertaking a new health care regimen. Never disregard professional medical advice or delay in seeking it because of something you have read in this book.

If you are experiencing a medical emergency, please call your local emergency number immediately.

The information provided in this book is provided "as is" without any representations or warranties, express or implied. To the fullest extent permitted by law, the author and the publisher exclude all representations, warranties, obligations, and liabilities arising out of or in connection with this book, including but not limited to warranties of merchantability, fitness for a particular purpose, and non-infringement of proprietary rights.

Limitation of Liability

In no event will the author or the publisher be liable for any direct, indirect, special, incidental, consequential, or punitive damages, including, without limitation, damages for loss of use, data, revenue, profits, business, or anticipated benefits, whether in action of contract, tort (including negligence), or otherwise, arising out of or in connection with the use of or reliance on any information, advice, or recommendations in this book.

By reading this book, you acknowledge that you are responsible for your own health decisions. Any application of the recommendations set forth in this book is at the reader's discretion and sole risk.

Copyright © 2023 Emrys Goldsworthy

All rights reserved

No part of this book may be reproduced, or stored in a retrieval system, or transmitted in any form or by any means, electronic, mechanical, photocopying, recording, or otherwise, without express written permission of the publisher.

Table of Contents

Preface: The Mysterious dance of the Vagus Nerve 1
Chapter 1   The Nervous System 3
Chapter 2   The Sympathetic Nervous System 11
Chapter 3   The Parasympathetic Nervous System 29
Chapter 4   The Vagus Nerve 35
Chapter 5   The Vagus Nerve and the Lungs. 45
Chapter 6   The Vagus Nerve and the Heart 51
Chapter 7   The Vagus Nerve and Swallowing 57
Chapter 8   The Vagus Nerve and Speech. 63
Chapter 9   The Vagus Nerve and the Oesophagus 69
Chapter 10   The Vagus Nerve and the Stomach 73
Chapter 11   The Vagus Nerve and the Small Intestines 79
Chapter 12   The Vagus Nerve and the Liver. 85
Chapter 13   The Vagus Nerve and the Gallbladder 91
Chapter 14   The Vagus Nerve and the Large Intestine 95
Chapter 15   The Vagus Nerve and the Kidneys 101
Chapter 16   The Vagus Nerve and the Bladder and Urethra. 105
Chapter 17   The Vagus Nerve and the Spleen 111
Chapter 18   The Vagus Nerve and the Pancreas 115
Chapter 19   The Vagus Nerve and the Male Reproductive System. 119
Chapter 20   The Vagus Nerve and the Female Reproductive System. 123
Chapter 21   The Vagus Nerve and The Brain 129

Chapter 22	The Cholinergic Anti-Inflammatory Pathway of the Vagus Nerve	135
Chapter 23	Vagus Nerve Dysfunction	139
Chapter 24	Causes of Vagus Nerve Dysfunction	147
Chapter 25	Vagus Nerve Assessment	155
Chapter 26	Treatment of the Vagus Nerve	161
Chapter 27	Optimising Vagal Tone	167
Chapter 28	Detoxification	185
Chapter 29	Epilepsy	195
Chapter 30	Atrial Fibrillation	201
Chapter 31	Migraine	205
Chapter 32	Depression	209
Chapter 33	Postural Orthostatic Tachycardia Syndrome	213
Chapter 34	Ehlers-Danlos Syndrome	217
Chapter 35	Mast Cell Activation Syndrome	225
Chapter 36	Is It All One disease?	231

Epilogue: The Harmonious Symphony of the Vagus Nerve ... 233

Preface:
The Mysterious Dance of the Vagus Nerve

Before you lies a voyage into one of the human body's most captivating tales, a tale spun through eons of evolution, painting a story of survival, adaptation, and profound connectivity: the story of the vagus nerve.

In ancient Latin, 'vagus' means 'wandering,' an apt description for this enigmatic cranial nerve. Its journey, stretching from the brain's depths to the heart and beyond the abdomen's confines, captures a microcosm of life's profound complexity. Yet, for many years, it remained in the background, a footnote in the grand annals of medical science. Today, however, its significance is unfolding, revealing secrets and possibilities that we once only dared to imagine.

This book seeks to be your compass as you navigate the complexities of the vagus nerve. Whether you are an aspiring medical student, a seasoned practitioner, or someone captivated by the wonders of human physiology, this exploration aims to offer insights that enrich your understanding and appreciation of the body.

Beyond just anatomical structures and physiological processes, you'll uncover the vagus nerve's role in emotions, mental well-being, and how our very thoughts can send ripples through its fibers, affecting our overall health.

It is a dance of science and mystery, where the known and the unknown twirl in tandem, beckoning us to join. So, as you turn the page, let yourself be pulled into the rhythm, the ebbs and flows, the highs and lows of the incredible journey of understanding the vagus nerve.

Welcome, dear reader, to the dance. Let's begin.

Chapter 1
The Nervous System

The grand tapestry of the human experience, interwoven with threads of sensation, motor responses, emotions, and cognition, finds its origin in the nervous system. Comprising billions of neurons, this intricate web forms the underpinning of our very existence.

Dichotomized into the central nervous system (CNS) and the peripheral nervous system (PNS), this structure forms a sophisticated network. While the CNS, encompassing the brain and spinal cord, functions as the primary command center, the PNS serves as the communication lines, connecting the CNS to every other part of our body.

A deeper dive into the PNS reveals two significant subdivisions: the somatic nervous system and the autonomic nervous system (ANS). While the former is involved in voluntary movements and the transference of sensory information to the CNS, the latter governs involuntary functions, making it integral to our body's automatic and often subconscious adjustments.

The Autonomic Nervous System

Integral to our existence, the ANS is a fascinating juxtaposition of precision and adaptability. Operating largely outside the realms of conscious thought, it seamlessly maintains a physiological equilibrium, ensuring that the body's internal environment remains stable amidst the ever-changing external landscape. Understanding its intricate mechanics offers profound insights into how humans navigate their daily lives, respond to stressors, and recuperate from exertions.

At a foundational level, the ANS is a network of neurons branching out from the spinal cord, reaching virtually every organ and tissue. It operates as a control system, functioning largely below the conscious radar, adjusting bodily processes such as heart rate, digestion, respiratory rate, pupillary response, and urination.

While its neurons originate in the brainstem and spinal cord, they extend far and wide, forming synapses with internal organs and ensuring that every physiological process is harmonized with the body's needs and environmental conditions.

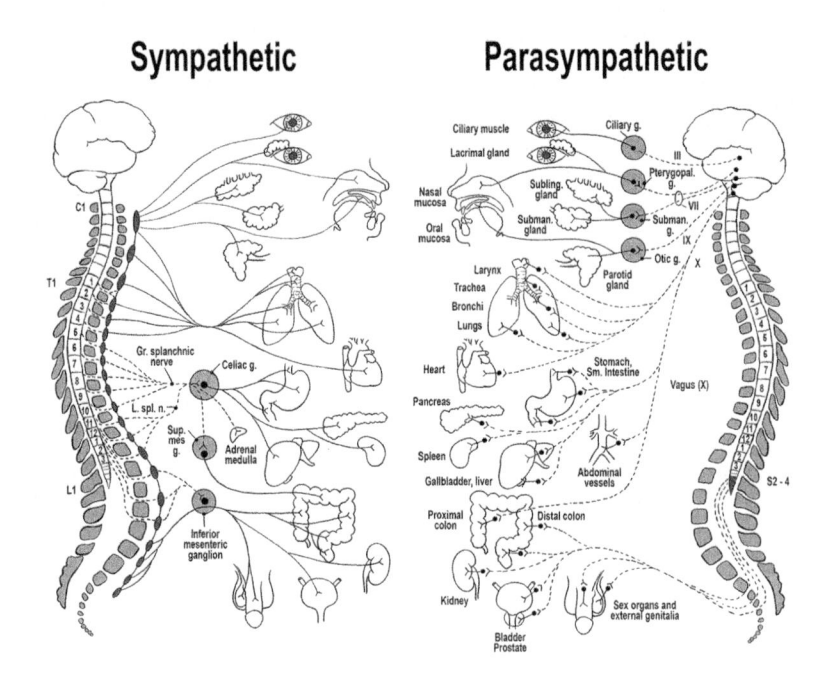

Functional Dichotomy

A standout feature of the ANS is its dichotomous division into the sympathetic and parasympathetic systems, each boasting a unique set of functions and responsibilities. This dual framework is emblematic of the body's need for balance. On one hand, the body requires mechanisms to confront or escape from immediate threats; on the other, it needs avenues to recuperate, restore energy, and heal.

The synergy between these systems ensures optimal functioning. Imagine the body as a finely-tuned orchestra, with each system playing a pivotal role. While the sympathetic system sounds the alarms and heightens the tempo during exigencies, the parasympathetic system introduces calming melodies, restoring balance and harmony.

Neurochemical Landscape

Driving the functions of the ANS is a complex neurochemical milieu. The transmission of impulses within this system is mediated by neurotransmitters, chemical messengers that convey signals between neurons and target tissues.

For instance, norepinephrine, released predominantly by the sympathetic fibers, accelerates the heart rate, increases blood flow to skeletal muscles, and heightens alertness. Conversely, acetylcholine, the primary neurotransmitter of the parasympathetic system, orchestrates a host of restorative functions, from slowing the heart rate to stimulating salivary gland secretion.

Interplay with the Endocrine System

The ANS does not operate in isolation. It continually interacts with the endocrine system, another pivotal regulatory system. This synergy is most evident in the adrenal medulla's response to stress—a direct outcome of sympathetic stimulation. In moments of acute stress, the adrenal glands secrete adrenaline, magnifying the sympathetic response and priming the body for action.

Feedback Mechanisms

Central to the ANS's efficient operation are feedback loops. These are mechanisms through which the system, after initiating a response, receives information about the effects of that response, and subsequently modulates its activity. For example, baroreceptors in blood vessels detect changes in blood pressure. If elevated, these receptors signal the brain to initiate parasympathetic responses to lower the pressure, thus ensuring homeostasis.

In essence, the ANS is a testament to nature's ingenuity—a system designed for both urgency and restoration, ensuring that the human body remains responsive and resilient in the face of life's myriad challenges. Its nuanced operations, though often imperceptible, are foundational to health and well-being.

Sympathetic versus Parasympathetic

The Dance of Dualities The human body, in its infinite wisdom, has constructed a dual system of internal checks and balances within the realm of the ANS. This ingenious design finds its most emblematic representation in the dichotomy of the sympathetic and parasympathetic nervous systems. Together, these systems form the dynamic duo governing our involuntary physiological processes, ensuring our survival, resilience, and recovery.

Sympathetic Nervous System (SNS): The Mobilizer Foundational Anatomy

Originating in the thoracolumbar region of the spinal cord, the sympathetic neurons extend their influence across a vast array of organs. From the dilation of pupils to the acceleration of heart rate, its neural tendrils weave through our body's fabric, ensuring readiness and reactivity.

Key Functions:
- Acceleration of Heart Rate and Blood Pressure: The SNS prepares the cardiovascular system for increased demand, ensuring oxygen-rich blood reaches vital organs and muscles expediently.

- Bronchial Dilation: To accommodate the heightened need for oxygen during stress or exertion, the bronchi of the lungs expand, allowing for increased air intake and oxygenation.

- Metabolic Activation: Mobilizing energy reserves, the SNS stimulates the release of glucose from liver stores, providing immediate energy sources for the body's needs.

- Inhibition of Non-essential Systems: Recognizing the primacy of immediate survival, the SNS temporarily suppresses systems not critical in crisis moments, like digestion and reproduction.

Parasympathetic Nervous System (PNS): The Restorer

With its craniosacral origin, the parasympathetic fibers emerge from the brainstem and the sacral segment of the spinal cord. The most prominent among them is the vagus nerve, influencing the heart, lungs, and digestive organs.

Key Functions:
- Heart Rate and Blood Pressure Reduction: Contrary to the SNS, the PNS orchestrates a decrease in heart rate and dilates blood vessels, promoting a restful state.
- Gastrointestinal Activation: Emphasizing rest and recuperation, the PNS stimulates salivation, gastric secretion, peristalsis, and other digestive processes, ensuring nutrient absorption and energy storage.
- Respiratory Modulation: The lungs undergo bronchoconstriction, reducing the respiratory rate and ensuring energy conservation.
- Reproductive and Urinary Systems: The PNS promotes activities related to growth, energy storage, and bodily maintenance, including reproductive functions and urination.

The Dynamic Interplay

The narrative of the SNS and PNS isn't one of stark antagonism, but rather of harmonious coordination. It's akin to the seamless transition between two seasoned dance partners, each aware of the other's movements, complementing each other to create a masterpiece of motion. While the SNS propels the body into action when urgency strikes, the PNS gracefully ushers in healing and recovery in moments of tranquility.

To truly appreciate the marvel that is human physiology, one need look no further than this intricate interplay. It's a delicate, dynamic equilibrium, ensuring that amid the cacophony of life's challenges, the body remains attuned, adaptive, and ever-evolving.

The Centrality of the Vagus Nerve

Embarking on an exploration of the PNS, one cannot sidestep the colossal influence of the vagus nerve. As the tenth cranial nerve, it originates from the medulla oblongata, situated in the brainstem, and forges a path through the neck, thorax, and abdomen, interfacing with vital organs such as the heart, lungs, and digestive tract.

Integral to the parasympathetic regulation, the vagus nerve orchestrates a multitude of functions. Its release of acetylcholine reduces heart rate, augments gastrointestinal peristalsis, facilitates nutrient absorption, and even impacts bronchoconstriction in the lungs. In juxtaposition to the SNS's alacrity, the vagus nerve heralds a return to restfulness and restoration.

Moreover, the delicate balance between the sympathetic and parasympathetic responses in the body owes much to the vagus nerve's modulation capabilities. While the 'fight or flight' response prepares the body to confront or flee from threats, the vagus nerve ensures that once the immediate danger subsides, the body reverts to its baseline, conserving energy and focusing on recuperation.

In conclusion, the human nervous system is a marvel of nature, intricately designed to maintain a delicate balance between action and rest, urgency and recovery. The interconnectedness of its various subdivisions, from the expansive reach of the CNS and PNS to the nuanced operations of the ANS, showcases the body's innate wisdom. The dance between the sympathetic and parasympathetic systems, governed by the vast influence of the vagus nerve, ensures that our body remains adaptive, responsive, and resilient. This intricate web of neurons, neurotransmitters, and feedback mechanisms not only facilitates our everyday experiences but is foundational to our very existence, health, and well-being. It stands as a testament to the complexities and wonders of human physiology, underscoring the importance of understanding and appreciating the systems that keep us alive and thriving.

References

1. Gage, N.M. and Baars, B., 2018. Fundamentals of Cognitive Neuroscience: A Beginner's Guide. 2nd edn. Elsevier.

2. Gibbons, C.H., 2019. Basics of autonomic nervous system function. Handb Clin Neurol, 160, pp.407-418. doi: 10.1016/B978-0-444-64032-1.00027-8. PMID: 31277865.

3. Purves, D., Augustine, G., Fitzpatrick, D., Hall, W., LaMantia, A., Mooney, R., Platt, M. and White, L. (eds.), 2017. Neuroscience: 6th Edition. Oxford University Press USA.

4. Squire, L., Berg, D., Bloom, F.E., du Lac, S., Ghosh, A. and Spitzer, N.C. (eds.), 2012. Fundamental Neuroscience. 4th edn. Elsevier.

5. Wehrwein, E.A., Orer, H.S. and Barman, S.M., 2016. Overview of the Anatomy, Physiology, and Pharmacology of the Autonomic Nervous System. Compr Physiol, 6(3), pp.1239-1278. doi: 10.1002/cphy.c150037. PMID: 27347892.

Chapter 2
The Sympathetic Nervous System

In our preceding exploration of the Autonomic Nervous System, we acquainted ourselves with the prime actors: the parasympathetic and sympathetic divisions. While the parasympathetic system drew our attention towards restoration and peace, the Sympathetic Nervous System (SNS) emerged as a compelling counterpoint — the embodiment of vigilance, action, and preparedness. Having brushed upon its overarching role in prompting the body's 'fight or flight' mechanics, this chapter intends to delve deeper. We aim to uncover the nuanced intricacies of the SNS, dissecting its anatomy, elucidating its functions, and appreciating its profound impact on our survival instincts and adaptability to external challenges.

Origins and Anatomy:
Delving Deeper into the Sympathetic Network

The SNS, often associated with the primal response of 'fight or flight', boasts an anatomical and functional intricacy that belies its seemingly straightforward mandate. This complexity is paramount to its adaptability, ensuring a nuanced response to a myriad of external stimuli.

Locus Coeruleus: A Command Center in the Pons
- Anatomical Location and Characteristics: The locus coeruleus, Latin for 'blue spot,' is situated bilaterally in the dorsal area of the pons, specifically in the lateral floor of the fourth ventricle within the brainstem. This nucleus is a component of the reticular formation and is proximal to the rostral end of the pons near its connection with the midbrain. Its unique bluish tint is due to the presence of neuromelanin, a specialized form of melanin found in nerve tissue.

- Role in Neurochemistry: This nucleus plays a significant role in the synthesis and release of the neurotransmitter noradrenaline. The locus coeruleus is the primary site in the brain responsible for the production of noradrenaline, serving as a central hub for neurochemical activities that have wide-ranging functional implications.

- Functional Characteristics: The locus coeruleus interacts directly with the SNS by sending descending projections to the spinal cord, which in turn affect sympathetic preganglionic neurons. This interaction enables the locus coeruleus to exert influence over various sympathetic responses, such as controlling heart rate, blood pressure, and pupil dilation.

- Cognitive Roles: Besides its involvement in sympathetic responses, the locus coeruleus has a broad range of functions related to cognition. It is key in the regulation of attention and wakefulness, affecting how attentively we respond to external stimuli. It also has a role in the sleep-wake cycle and can influence levels of wakefulness and arousal.

- Emotional Regulation: The nucleus is also implicated in the regulation of emotional responses. Its role in the release of noradrenaline amplifies the body's fight-or-flight response and enhances its ability to react to stressful or hazardous situations.

Summary: The locus coeruleus serves as a central hub in the brain, coordinating the functions of the SNS with higher-level cognitive and emotional processes. Its unique anatomical positioning and functional versatility make it pivotal in the integration and regulation of both physiological and cognitive activities. Understanding the locus coeruleus is essential for a comprehensive grasp of the SNS's operations and its interconnectedness with the brain's central nuclei.

Locus Coeruleus to Spinal Cord: Detailed Pathways
- Noradrenergic Neurons: The locus coeruleus contains specialized neurons that predominantly release the neurotransmitter noradrenaline. These neurons send their axons down the brainstem

and into the spinal cord via several descending tracts, most notably the dorsolateral and ventrolateral funiculi.

- Intermediolateral Cell Column (IML): These descending axons from the locus coeruleus make synaptic connections primarily within the intermediolateral cell column of the spinal cord. This is a specialized group of neurons located in the lateral horn of the spinal cord's gray matter, specifically between the T1 and L2 segments. The IML serves as a crucial interface for sympathetic outflow, housing the cell bodies of sympathetic preganglionic neurons.

- Signal Transmission: The locus coeruleus modulates the activity of these sympathetic preganglionic neurons by releasing noradrenaline. This neurotransmitter binds to adrenergic receptors on these neurons, either enhancing or suppressing their activity depending on the receptor type and the context of the neural input.

Spinal Cord to Sympathetic Ganglia: The Neural Relay

- White and Grey Rami Communicantes: Rami communicantes are small nerve branches that act as liaisons between the spinal nerves and sympathetic ganglia. Each spinal nerve is connected to its corresponding ganglion by two types of rami communicantes: white and gray. The white rami communicantes are preganglionic fibers that carry signals from the spinal cord to the ganglia. These fibers are myelinated, giving them their white appearance. In contrast, the gray rami communicantes are postganglionic fibers, which are usually unmyelinated and carry signals from the ganglia back to the spinal nerves.

- Functional Characteristics: The color distinction between the white and gray rami is not merely aesthetic; it carries functional implications. The myelin sheath around the white rami acts as an insulator, speeding up the transmission of nerve impulses. This is particularly important in the context of the SNS, where quick response times are often crucial. For instance, when faced with danger, the body doesn't have the luxury of time; it needs to react quickly to either 'fight' or take 'flight.'

Ganglia: Neuronal Hubs of Targeted Action

Ganglia are clusters of neurons found in two parallel chains that run on either side of the vertebral column. Each ganglion houses neuronal cell bodies and is a mini-hub where synaptic connections occur. The sympathetic ganglia are often categorized into cervical, thoracic, lumbar, and sacral regions, aligning with the vertebral segments they serve. These classifications serve as landmarks, aiding in the identification of their specific roles and territories.

The abdominal and pelvic organs, vital as they are, demand their own dedicated regulatory hubs. Enter the collateral or prevertebral ganglia. Clustered around major arteries like the aorta, these ganglia, including the celiac, superior mesenteric, and inferior mesenteric ganglia, are pivotal. They are the crossroads where spinal instructions translate into tangible changes in organ function, from the churning of the stomach to the filtration prowess of the kidneys.

- Functional Characteristics: When a stimulus triggers the SNS, preganglionic neurons emerge from the spinal cord and synapse with the neurons in the corresponding ganglia. This targeted synapsing helps the body activate or inhibit specific functions like heart rate increase or dilation of pupils, based on the nature of the stimulus.

- Target Tissues: When a stimulus is detected, the preganglionic neurons housed in the spinal cord send an urgent signal through the white rami to the corresponding ganglia. Once the message is processed and the appropriate response is determined, postganglionic neurons transmit the signal via the gray rami. Each postganglionic neuron may send its axon to specific target tissues, enabling a very targeted sympathetic response. The signal can reach a variety of peripheral targets, ranging from blood vessels and heart muscle to glands and smooth muscle in various organs.

- Summary: The sympathetic chain, comprising ganglia and rami communicantes, serves as a sophisticated vertebral odyssey that houses and transports crucial neuronal signals. It acts as both a structural and functional bridge between the spinal cord and the rest of the body, ensuring quick, targeted responses to external stimuli. Through its anatomical arrangement and functional capabilities, the sympathetic chain stands as a testament to the complexity and efficiency of the body's internal communication systems.

Interplay Between the SNS and the HPA Axis

The Hypothalamic-Pituitary-Adrenal (HPA) axis represents one of the most critical neuroendocrine systems in the human body, responsible for regulating a wide range of bodily functions, including stress response, metabolism, immune function, and circadian rhythms. Understanding the HPA axis is pivotal to appreciating its synergistic relationships with other systems, including the SNS. This axis consists of three primary components: the hypothalamus, the pituitary gland, and the adrenal glands, each with its unique roles and functions.

The Hypothalamus: Located in the diencephalon region of the brain, the hypothalamus serves as the primary regulatory hub for various physiological functions and behaviors. Its role in the HPA axis begins with the sensing of stressors—be they physical, emotional, or cognitive. In response to such stimuli, the hypothalamus secretes corticotropin-releasing hormone (CRH), which acts as the initial messenger in this hormonal cascade.

The Pituitary Gland: Situated just below the hypothalamus, the pituitary gland is often termed the "master gland" due to its broad spectrum of hormonal regulatory functions. Within the context of the HPA axis, the anterior portion of the pituitary gland is of prime interest. Upon receiving CRH from the hypothalamus, the anterior pituitary secretes adrenocorticotropic hormone (ACTH). This hormone travels through the bloodstream to act on the adrenal glands, which are situated atop the kidneys.

The Adrenal Medulla: A Unique Nexus of the SNS The human body is a masterpiece of coordination and synergy, and the adrenal medulla stands as a testament to this intricate design. As a core component of the adrenal glands, which perch atop our kidneys like protective guardians, the adrenal medulla serves a pivotal role in our sympathetic response. But what sets it apart from other sympathetic endpoints, and why is it of such profound importance?

Role in SNS: The adrenal medulla is integral to the "fight-or-flight" response mediated by the SNS. Upon sympathetic activation, the adrenal medulla rapidly secretes catecholamines into the bloodstream.

Role in HPA Axis: Conversely, the adrenal cortex's role in the HPA axis involves a slower, more sustained response to stress. Triggered by ACTH from the pituitary gland, the adrenal cortex secretes cortisol, which has broad systemic effects. These include the modulation of metabolism (through gluconeogenesis and lipolysis), suppression of immune responses, and the regulation of blood pressure. Cortisol secretion follows a circadian rhythm and serves longer-term adaptive functions compared to the rapid actions of catecholamines.

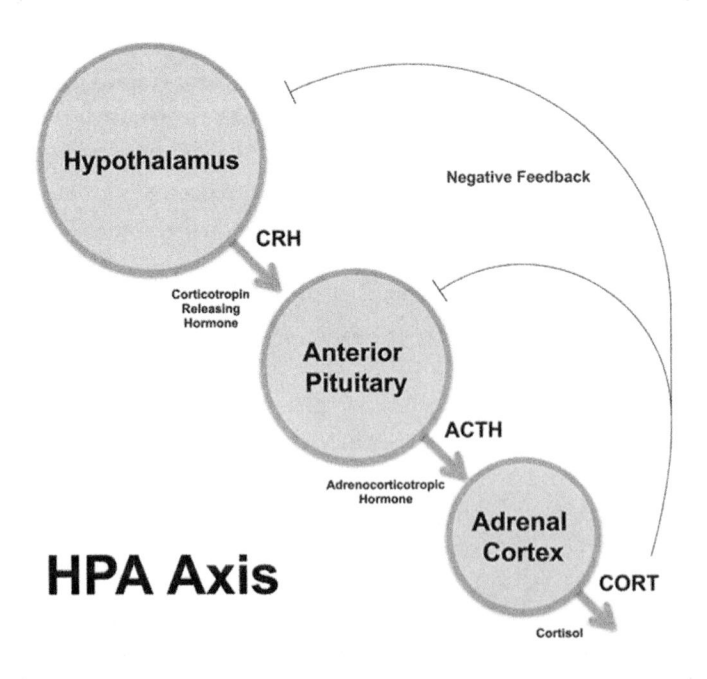

Comparative Summary: The adrenal medulla and adrenal cortex play complementary roles in managing stress, each with distinct timing, hormone secretion, regulatory mechanisms, and systemic impact. Acting rapidly within seconds to minutes in response to acute stress, the adrenal medulla is directly stimulated by sympathetic preganglionic neurons to secrete catecholamines, which prepare the body for immediate physical activity. In contrast, the adrenal cortex has a slower onset of action but sustains its effects for a more extended period, producing cortisol for prolonged stress adaptation through a hormonal cascade involving the hypothalamus and pituitary gland. While catecholamines focus on priming the body for quick action, cortisol exerts broader, more modulatory effects on various physiological processes, including immune suppression and metabolic regulation.

Embryological Origins: Unlike the rest of the adrenal gland, the adrenal medulla originates from the neural crest cells, a population of embryonic cells that also gives rise to neurons of the SNS. This shared lineage intimately ties the adrenal medulla to the SNS, rendering it a specialized endpoint.

Neuroendocrine Hybrid: The adrenal medulla is a unique blend of neural and endocrine characteristics. While it's innervated by preganglionic sympathetic fibers, it doesn't synapse with postganglionic neurons as in typical sympathetic pathways. Instead, chromaffin cells, the primary cell type in the medulla, act as modified postganglionic neurons. Upon stimulation, they don't transmit nerve impulses; they release hormones directly into the bloodstream.

The Catecholamine Factory: Over 80% of the body's adrenaline (epinephrine) and a significant proportion of noradrenaline (norepinephrine) are synthesized, stored, and released by the adrenal medulla. In response to acute stress, these catecholamines flood the bloodstream within seconds, ensuring a swift and comprehensive 'fight or flight' response.

Regulatory Mechanisms: The secretion of catecholamines isn't random; it's meticulously regulated. The splanchnic nerve, which innervates the adrenal medulla, transmits signals based on inputs from the brain, especially regions like the hypothalamus. Thus, the adrenal medulla acts as a bridge, translating neural inputs into endocrine outputs.

Rapid Response, Broad Impact: Because the adrenal medulla releases its hormones directly into the bloodstream, its effects are both rapid and widespread. From increasing heart rate to mobilizing energy reserves, the influence of adrenal catecholamines is far-reaching, preparing nearly every organ and system for impending action.

Resilience and Adaptation: While the adrenal medulla is primed for quick responses, it's also adaptable. Chronic stress or recurrent acute stress can alter its functional dynamics, leading to changes in catecholamine synthesis, storage, and release. This plasticity ensures that the organ remains responsive and relevant to the body's changing needs.

In essence, the adrenal medulla is more than just an endpoint of the SNS. It's a specialized neuroendocrine hub, serving as a crucial bridge between our nervous and endocrine systems. By translating neural signals into hormonal cascades, it ensures that our 'fight or flight' response is both swift and systemic, preparing us for the myriad challenges that life throws our way.

Physiological Responses: The All-Encompassing Role of Adrenaline and Noradrenaline

In the face of perceived danger or acute stress, the body's immediate task is to prepare for action, be it to confront the threat ('fight') or to evade it ('flight'). This rapid, holistic adjustment is primarily orchestrated by the sympathetic release of two catecholamines: adrenaline (also known as epinephrine) and noradrenaline (norepinephrine). Their effects permeate every corner of our physiology, ensuring that we are optimally primed to respond to the crisis. Here, we delineate these manifold effects, highlighting the vast reach of these potent molecules:

Cardiovascular System
- Heart Rate and Contractility: Both catecholamines increase the heart's rate and contractile force, ensuring increased cardiac output.
- Vascular Tone: While they generally cause vasoconstriction to elevate blood pressure, there's selective vasodilation in skeletal muscles,

supporting potential physical action.
- Blood Flow Redistribution: There's a preferential diversion of blood towards essential organs like the heart and brain and away from less crucial sites during stress, such as the gastrointestinal system.

Respiratory System:
- Bronchodilation: Both chemicals prompt the bronchioles to expand, ensuring optimal oxygen intake.
- Increased Respiratory Rate: This ensures a faster oxygen-carbon dioxide exchange to sustain heightened metabolic demands.

Metabolic Responses:
- Glycogenolysis and Gluconeogenesis: The liver breaks down glycogen to glucose and also synthesizes glucose, ensuring ample energy supply.
- Lipolysis: Fat cells break down triglycerides to release fatty acids as an additional energy source.
- Metabolic Rate: The overall metabolic rate rises, elevating body temperature.

Musculoskeletal System:
- Muscle Preparation: There's increased blood flow to skeletal muscles, heightened glucose uptake, and an elevated readiness for contraction.

Neurological Effects:
- Alertness and Focus: Both neurotransmitters elevate cerebral alertness and the ability to focus on the task at hand.
- Pupil Dilation: This ensures optimal light intake and clearer vision of potential threats or escape routes.

Endocrine System:
- Inhibition of Insulin: Reduced insulin release promotes hyperglycemia, providing more glucose as an energy substrate.
- Stimulation of Renin: This initiates the renin-angiotensin-aldosterone system, further supporting blood pressure elevation.

Gastrointestinal and Renal Systems:
- Gastrointestinal Mobility: There's a marked reduction, as digestion isn't a priority during acute stress.
- Bladder Relaxation: The body postpones the need to void.
- Renal Blood Flow: Generally reduced to prioritize other organs, but with an increased release of renin to support blood pressure regulation.

Integumentary System:
- Sweat Production: Elevated, preparing the body for potential overheating from action.
- Piloerection: Hair stands on end (often termed "goosebumps"), a vestigial response.

Immune System:
- Short-term Boost: Initially, there's a mobilization of immune cells, but prolonged stress can suppress immunity.

Reproductive System:
- Inhibition: Acute stress often suppresses reproductive function, including reduced libido and, in prolonged scenarios, can disrupt menstrual cycles.

This all-encompassing cascade, stemming from the release of adrenaline and noradrenaline, transforms our physiology almost instantaneously, optimizing our body for the crisis at hand. This physiological symphony, though demanding, is testament to the body's remarkable ability to adapt and confront challenges head-on.

The Sympathetic Balance: Beyond the Stress Paradigm

Often, when one mentions the SNS, it conjures images of high-adrenaline situations — escaping danger, facing confrontation, or merely the stress of a looming deadline. Yet, to pigeonhole the SNS solely within this frame is to misunderstand its all-encompassing nature. Far from just orchestrating 'fight or flight' reactions, the SNS is a tireless sentinel, constantly at work to ensure our body's equilibrium.

Blood Pressure Regulation: Even in the absence of overt stress, the SNS maintains a certain degree of vascular tone, ensuring that blood pressure doesn't fall too low. It ensures that blood consistently reaches all tissues, from the oxygen-thirsty brain to the nutrient-demanding muscles.

Baroreceptor Reflex: This elegant feedback system involves stretch receptors in major vessels like the carotid artery. Should they detect a dip in pressure, they communicate with the brain, prompting an increase in sympathetic outflow, which tightens vessels and elevates the heart rate.

Temperature Regulation: When we're cold, the SNS instigates a series of events leading to heat generation. This includes increasing metabolic activities in cells, especially brown adipose tissue, and inducing shivering.

Vasoconstriction: Another tactic in the cold is to reduce blood flow to the skin, minimizing heat loss. The SNS prompts vessels in the skin to constrict, ensuring our core remains warm.

Metabolic Oversight: Even outside stressful scenarios, the SNS modulates glucose levels. It promotes the breakdown of glycogen in the liver, ensuring that glucose is continually supplied to vital tissues.

Lipolysis: The SNS encourages fat cells to release fatty acids into the bloodstream, providing an energy source for cells. This isn't just vital during physical exertion; it's part of routine energy regulation.

Gastrointestinal Harmony: While stress is known to slow digestion, the SNS, in its quieter moments, helps coordinate regular bowel movements and the churning of stomach contents, ensuring efficient digestion and nutrient absorption.

Pulmonary Equilibrium: Even outside of the classic 'fight or flight' situations where we might need more oxygen, the SNS subtly modulates bronchial diameter, ensuring optimal air passage for routine respiration.

Renal Balance: A critical aspect of blood pressure and fluid regulation, the SNS stimulates the kidneys to release renin, a precursor in a pathway that eventually leads to the conservation of sodium and water.

Musculoskeletal Readiness: Even when we're not consciously moving, our muscles maintain a certain degree of tension, or tone. This readiness, ensuring we can spring into action if needed, is modulated in part by the SNS.

In summation, the SNS is not a mere responder to crises; it is a vigilant guardian of our physiological balance. By ceaselessly adjusting and recalibrating various parameters, it ensures that the vast, interconnected machinery of our body remains in harmony, regardless of external challenges. Far from just reacting to stress, the SNS is intrinsically woven into the very fabric of our daily existence.

Pathological Implications: The Perils of Sympathetic Overdrive

While the SNS is indispensable for maintaining homeostasis and responding to challenges, its chronic overactivity or dysregulation can have significant pathological implications. An understanding of these is essential, not just from a clinical perspective, but also for appreciating the fine balance our bodies continually strive to achieve.

Cardiovascular Complications:

Hypertension: One of the most recognized complications of sustained sympathetic activation is elevated blood pressure. Over time, this can strain the heart, damage blood vessels, and increase the risk of heart attacks, strokes, and kidney diseases.

Cardiac Hypertrophy: The heart, when persistently overworked due to high SNS activity, may enlarge – a condition called hypertrophy. This can lead to heart failure, arrhythmias, and other complications.

Atherosclerosis: Chronic stress and sustained sympathetic activity have been linked to the acceleration of atherosclerosis, the buildup of plaques in arteries, which can result in heart attacks and strokes.

Metabolic Derangements:

Insulin Resistance and Type 2 Diabetes: Over time, chronic sympathetic activation can lead to insulin resistance, a precursor for Type 2 diabetes. This may occur due to the consistent mobilization of glucose and fats in the bloodstream.

Weight Gain and Obesity: Chronic stress and heightened SNS activity can increase appetite and lead to accumulation of visceral fat, a type of fat linked to numerous health risks.

Gastrointestinal Disruptions:

Stress Ulcers: Excessive sympathetic activity can reduce blood flow to the stomach lining, making it susceptible to the corrosive action of stomach acids. This can lead to the formation of ulcers.

Irritable Bowel Syndrome (IBS): IBS, characterized by a mix of abdominal pain, bloating, constipation, and diarrhea, can be exacerbated by chronic stress and heightened SNS activation.

Neurological and Cognitive Implications:

Anxiety and Panic Disorders: Persistent sympathetic overdrive can manifest as chronic anxiety, and in acute surges, can lead to panic attacks.

Insomnia and Sleep Disturbances: Elevated SNS activity, especially during nighttime, can disrupt the sleep-wake cycle, preventing restorative sleep and leading to chronic fatigue and cognitive impairments.

Immune System Dysfunction:

Immune Suppression: Chronic stress and SNS activation can suppress the immune response, making the body more susceptible to infections. Additionally, wounds may heal slower, and vaccinations might be less effective.

Inflammation: Paradoxically, while suppressing some immune functions, chronic stress might also lead to systemic inflammation, increasing the risk for several chronic diseases, including cardiovascular diseases and certain cancers.

Endocrine and Reproductive Alterations:

Hypothalamic-Pituitary-Adrenal (HPA) Axis Dysregulation: Chronic stress can dysregulate the HPA axis, leading to disorders like Cushing's syndrome or Addison's disease.

Reproductive Dysfunction: Chronic SNS overactivity can lead to menstrual irregularities in women, reduced libido in both genders, and even erectile dysfunction in men.

Musculoskeletal Issues:

Tension Headaches and Migraines: Prolonged muscle tension, especially in the neck and scalp regions, can lead to tension headaches. Moreover, migraines can be triggered or exacerbated by chronic stress.

Muscle Atrophy and Weakness: Constantly elevated stress hormones can lead to protein breakdown and muscle wasting over time.

Cortisol Resistance Due to Chronic Stress

Cortisol resistance is a physiological phenomenon that emerges in the context of chronic stress exposure, where tissues become desensitized to the effects of cortisol, the primary glucocorticoid hormone released by the adrenal glands. Normally, cortisol plays a pivotal role in various physiological processes, including immune response modulation, metabolic regulation, and stress adaptation. However, chronic stress can lead to disruptions in cortisol signaling and receptor sensitivity, resulting in diminished responsiveness to cortisol's regulatory effects.

Mechanism of Cortisol Resistance

Cortisol typically exerts its effects by binding to intracellular glucocorticoid receptors (GRs), which then translocate to the nucleus and modulate the transcription of specific genes. In the context of cortisol resistance, several mechanisms have been proposed:

- Downregulation of Receptors: Chronic exposure to high cortisol levels may lead to a decrease in the number of available GRs, effectively reducing tissue sensitivity to cortisol.

- Impaired Receptor Binding: Structural modifications in GRs could hinder effective binding, making it more difficult for cortisol to exert its effects.

- Intracellular Signaling Alterations: Post-translational modifications of intracellular signaling molecules could disrupt the transduction pathways that cortisol usually activates.

- Competitive Inhibition: Inflammatory cytokines or other hormones may competitively inhibit GRs, thus reducing cortisol's effectiveness.

Physiological Consequences

- Immunological Effects: One of cortisol's main functions is to regulate immune responses. Cortisol resistance can lead to unregulated inflammation and potentially contribute to the development of autoimmune or inflammatory diseases.

- Metabolic Impact: Cortisol plays a vital role in glucose metabolism and insulin sensitivity. Resistance to cortisol could contribute to metabolic syndrome, insulin resistance, and increased cardiovascular risk.

- Mental Health: Chronic stress and cortisol resistance are also associated with various mental health issues, including anxiety, depression, and increased susceptibility to stress-induced disorders.

- Endocrine Disruption: Cortisol resistance can disrupt the feedback loop within the HPA axis, leading to elevated or erratic cortisol levels, which could further exacerbate physiological imbalances.

Clinical Relevance

Understanding cortisol resistance is crucial for developing effective treatments for a host of stress-related disorders, including chronic fatigue syndrome, fibromyalgia, and various anxiety and depressive disorders. It's also pertinent in the management of autoimmune diseases and conditions with a significant inflammatory component.

Conclusion: The Vigilant Sentinel – A Tribute to the SNS

As we close this exploration into the SNS, it is essential to acknowledge and marvel at its intricate design and invaluable function. More than just a biological system, the SNS emerges as a vigilant sentinel, ceaselessly overseeing and safeguarding our body's physiological landscape.

Guardian of Homeostasis:

At its core, the SNS is a protector. Whether it's rapidly responding to immediate threats or subtly tweaking internal processes, its central objective remains unwavering: the preservation of balance and homeostasis. The myriad physiological adjustments it orchestrates, often behind the scenes, underpin the essence of life itself.

Responder to the External World:

The SNS serves as our primary interface with the dynamic and unpredictable external environment. Every stimulus, whether it's the chill of winter air or the thrill of a roller coaster, elicits a calibrated SNS response, ensuring we remain attuned and adaptable to external shifts.

In Sync with Modern Challenges:

Evolutionarily speaking, our SNS was fashioned to address primal threats – predators, famine, and natural disasters. Yet, it's a testament to its flexibility that it now grapples with the stresses of modern life, from traffic jams to tight work deadlines.

Synergy with Other Systems:

While it stands as a formidable entity on its own, the true prowess of the SNS shines when it collaborates with other physiological systems. Whether it's the dance with the parasympathetic nervous system to maintain cardiac rhythm or its partnership with the endocrine system to ensure metabolic harmony, the SNS is a team player.

A Call for Respect and Care: Understanding the magnitude of the SNS's role imparts a profound responsibility. Modern lifestyles often push our sympathetic machinery into overdrive, leading to numerous health implications. Recognizing these challenges, we must be proactive in managing stress, seeking balance, and fostering environments that honor our biological heritage.

Forward into the Future: As medical science progresses, we are continually uncovering the deeper nuances of the SNS. Its role in illnesses, its interaction with emerging technologies, and its response to novel stressors like space travel or virtual realities remain burgeoning areas of research. With every new revelation, the depth and breadth of our sentinel's role expand, solidifying its stature as a cornerstone of human physiology.

In retrospection, the SNS emerges not just as a component of our anatomy but as a testament to the intricate and awe-inspiring nature of life. As we journey forward, let's carry with us a profound respect for this vigilant sentinel, recognizing its tireless service and striving always to uphold the delicate balance it so valiantly protects.

References

1. Baars, B. and Gage, N. M. 2018. Fundamentals of Cognitive Neuroscience: A Beginner's Guide, 2nd ed. Elsevier.

2. Borsook, D., Haas, A., Freeman, R. and Adler, G. 2022. 'Stress, hypoglycemia, and the autonomic nervous system', Auton Neurosci, 240, pp. 102983. doi: 10.1016/j.autneu.2022.102983.

3. Brookes, S., Hibberd, T., Yew, W. P., Spencer, N. J. and Costa, M. 2022. 'Enteric Control of the Sympathetic Nervous System', Adv Exp Med Biol, 1383, pp. 89-103. doi: 10.1007/978-3-031-05843-1_9.

4. Domingos, A. I., Martinez-Sanchez, N., Sweeney, O., Sidarta-Oliveira, D., Caron, A. and Stanley, S. A. 2022. 'The sympathetic nervous system in the 21st century: Neuroimmune interactions in metabolic homeostasis and obesity', Neuron, 110(21), pp. 3597-3626. doi: 10.1016/j.neuron.2022.10.017.

5. Kuruvilla, R., Scott-Solomon, E. and Boehm, E. 2021. 'The sympathetic nervous system in development and disease', Nat Rev Neurosci, 22(11), pp. 685-702. doi: 10.1038/s41583-021-00523-y.

6. Platt, M., Purves, D., Augustine, G., Mooney, R., LaMantia, A., Fitzpatrick, D., Hall, W. and White, L. (eds.) 2017. Neuroscience: 6th Edition. Oxford University Press USA.

7. Pongratz, G. and Straub, R. H. 2023. 'Rolle des sympathischen Nervensystems bei chronischen Entzündungen [Role of the sympathetic nervous system in chronic inflammation]', Z Rheumatol, 82(6), pp. 451-461. doi: 10.1007/s00393-023-01387-6.

Chapter 3
The Parasympathetic Nervous System

The intricate tapestry of the human nervous system intricately governs everything from our most deliberate actions to the subtlest of internal processes. A particularly fascinating weave in this vast system is the parasympathetic nervous system (PNS). Unlike its counterpart, the sympathetic system, which propels the body into action during moments of stress, the PNS has earned the moniker "rest and digest" due to its essential role in facilitating processes that conserve and restore energy.

The PNS doesn't just operate in the background; it's at the forefront of ensuring our body's homeostasis. It carefully regulates functions ranging from slowing the heart rate after a strenuous activity to aiding in the digestive process after a meal. By actively reducing the "alert" signals and promoting states of calm, the PNS helps us recuperate and refresh, ensuring our bodies are ready for subsequent activities.

In this chapter, we will delve deep into the heart of the PNS, exploring its structure, functions, and significance in maintaining our physiological equilibrium. This exploration will elucidate the silent, yet powerful, forces at work that allow our bodies to recover, rejuvenate, and remain in balance.

Anatomy and Neural Pathways of the PNS

Understanding the PNS's full breadth requires a deep dive into its anatomical structure and the neural pathways it navigates. This intricate web of pathways, stemming from the brain and spinal cord, regulates some of our most vital physiological processes.

THE VAGUS NERVE

Craniosacral Origin:

The PNS, often termed the "craniosacral system", originates from the brainstem and the sacral portion of the spinal cord. Specifically, its fibers arise from the brain's cranial nerves and the S2 to S4 sacral spinal segments.

1. Cranial Components:

- Oculomotor Nerve (CN III): This nerve manages the constriction of the pupil and the lens's accommodation in the eye. It originates from the Edinger-Westphal nucleus and projects to the ciliary ganglion, which further sends fibers to the eye's intrinsic muscles.

- Facial Nerve (CN VII): It has parasympathetic fibers responsible for stimulating the lacrimal glands (tear production) and salivary glands. The superior salivatory nucleus gives rise to these fibers, which project to both the pterygopalatine and submandibular ganglia.

- Glossopharyngeal Nerve (CN IX): This nerve controls the parotid salivary gland. Its fibers originate from the inferior salivatory nucleus, projecting to the otic ganglion, which in turn sends fibers to the parotid gland.

- Vagus Nerve (CN X): The most extensive parasympathetic cranial nerve, the vagus nerve, originates from the dorsal nucleus of the vagus and the nucleus ambiguus. This nerve innervates many organs, including the heart, lungs, and most of the digestive tract. It plays roles in heart rate moderation, peristalsis stimulation in the gut, bronchoconstriction in the lungs, and various other functions.

2. Sacral Components:

The sacral portion of the PNS emerges from the second, third, and fourth sacral spinal cord segments (S2, S3, and S4). These preganglionic fibers project to the pelvic ganglia. From here, postganglionic fibers innervate a range of pelvic organs:

- Urinary bladder: Promotes bladder contraction and relaxation of the internal urethral sphincter for urination.

- Rectum: Modulates activity for defecation.

- Sexual organs: Involvement in erection (vasodilation) and lubrication.

Neurotransmitters and Receptors:
- Acetylcholine: Both the preganglionic and postganglionic neurons of the PNS release acetylcholine as their primary neurotransmitter.
- Nicotinic Receptors: Found on the cell bodies and dendrites of all postganglionic neurons (both sympathetic and parasympathetic). Acetylcholine from preganglionic neurons binds to these receptors.
- Muscarinic Receptors: These are found on the target tissues innervated by postganglionic parasympathetic fibers. Acetylcholine from these fibers interacts with these receptors to induce various physiological effects.

Ganglia in the PNS:

While the sympathetic system's ganglia often lie far from the target organs (forming a chain beside the vertebral column), the parasympathetic ganglia are usually located close to or within the target organs themselves. This closeness allows for a more localized and specific response.

Conclusion: The anatomy and neural pathways of the PNS showcase a beautifully orchestrated system, fine-tuned for specificity and restoration. Its intricate connections, spanning from the cranial structures down to the sacral spinal cord, are quintessential in maintaining homeostasis and ensuring our body's calm and recuperative states.

The Parasympathetic Equilibrium: Beyond the Restorative Facade

When discussing the PNS, many think of relaxation, rejuvenation, and a slowdown of bodily activities. However, the PNS is much more than just a controller of the "rest and digest" states; it's actively involved in numerous functions that maintain and restore the body's equilibrium.

Cardiovascular System:
  a. Heart Rate Reduction: The PNS slows down the heart rate through the release of acetylcholine, conserving energy and maintaining a

steady pace for the heart.

  b. Vasodilation: In certain vessels, the PNS promotes dilation, allowing for increased blood flow to specific organs or regions.

Digestive System:
  a. Salivation: It stimulates salivary glands to produce saliva, starting the digestion process.
  b. Enzyme Secretion: It enhances the secretion of digestive enzymes from various glands to aid in digestion.
  c. Peristalsis Stimulation: The PNS actively promotes the rhythmic movement of the intestines, helping in the movement of food and waste.
  d. Gastric Juice Production: It stimulates the stomach lining to produce gastric juices essential for digestion.
  e. Bile Release: It regulates the gallbladder's release of bile into the small intestine, aiding in fat digestion.

Ocular System:
  a. Pupillary Constriction: The PNS helps in narrowing the pupils in response to high light intensity.
  b. Lens Accommodation: Adjusts the lens shape for near vision, ensuring clear focus.

Urinary System:
  a. Bladder Contraction: Promotes the contraction of the bladder's detrusor muscle, allowing urination.
  b. Relaxation of the Internal Urethral Sphincter: This facilitates the release of urine.

Respiratory System:
  a. Bronchoconstriction: The PNS narrows the bronchi in the lungs during calm states, maintaining a consistent airflow.
  b. Secretion Stimulation: Enhances secretion within respiratory

passages, aiding in humidifying and filtering the air.

Reproductive System:
   a. Erection in Males: Promotes vasodilation in the erectile tissues, allowing for sexual arousal.
   b. Lubrication in Females: Stimulates the secretion of lubricating fluids during arousal.

Endocrine System:
   a. Pancreatic Function: Modulates the release of digestive enzymes and bicarbonate from the pancreas.

Integumentary System:
   a. Promotion of Glandular Activities: In specific scenarios, the PNS can influence certain glandular secretions in the skin, though its role here is not as dominant as the sympathetic system.

Lacrimal System:
   a. Tear Production: Stimulates the lacrimal glands to produce tears, ensuring the eyes remain moist and debris-free.

Musculoskeletal System:
   a. Muscle Energy Conservation: By slowing down the heart rate and respiration during periods of rest, the PNS ensures muscles have a continuous supply of oxygen and nutrients without overexertion.

In summation, the PNS is intricately interwoven into the fabric of our physiology. Its roles span across systems and functions, constantly working to ensure restoration, maintenance, and balance. Far from just being a passive system of relaxation, the PNS exemplifies the intricate choreography that goes into keeping our bodies in equilibrium.

References:

1. Augustine, G., Purves, D., Fitzpatrick, D., Mooney, R., LaMantia, A., Hall, W., Platt, M. and White, L. (eds.) 2017. Neuroscience: 6th Edition. Oxford University Press USA.

2. Baars, B. and Gage, N. M. 2018. Fundamentals of Cognitive Neuroscience: A Beginner's Guide, 2nd ed. Elsevier.

3. Berg, D., Squire, L., Bloom, F. E., du Lac, S., Ghosh, A. and Spitzer, N. C. (eds.) 2012. Fundamental Neuroscience, 4th ed. Elsevier.

4. Khan, A. A., Lip, G. Y. H., and Shantsila, A. 2019. 'Heart rate variability in atrial fibrillation: The balance between sympathetic and parasympathetic nervous system', Eur J Clin Invest, 49(11), e13174. doi: 10.1111/eci.13174.

5. Ramchandra, R. and Shanks, J. 2021. 'Angiotensin II and the Cardiac Parasympathetic Nervous System in Hypertension', Int J Mol Sci, 22(22), 12305. doi: 10.3390/ijms222212305.

6. Tadi, P. and Tindle, J. 2022. 'Neuroanatomy, Parasympathetic Nervous System', In: StatPearls [Internet]. Treasure Island (FL): StatPearls Publishing; 2023 Jan.

Chapter 4
The Vagus Nerve

The vagus nerve (cranial nerve X) is one of the most complex cranial nerves, given its widespread distribution and varied functions. It possesses several nuclei and ganglia, which house the nerve's cell bodies. These act as stations for motor output and sensory feedback.

Anatomy: Nuclei of the Vagus Nerve

Dorsal Motor Nucleus:
- Location: The dorsal motor nucleus is located deep in the medulla, near the midline and close to the floor of the fourth ventricle. It's positioned medially to the solitary nucleus and tract.
- Function: It provides parasympathetic preganglionic fibers to the heart, lungs, and most of the digestive tract. These fibers exit the CNS and synapse on postganglionic neurons in various organs, influencing functions like heart rate and gastrointestinal motility.

Nucleus Ambiguus:
- Location: The nucleus ambiguus is situated within the medulla oblongata, lying dorsally (towards the back) to the inferior olivary nucleus and in the retro-olivary region. It is situated laterally to the dorsal motor nucleus of the vagus nerve.
- Function: Supplies branchiomotor fibers to certain muscles of the pharynx, larynx, and the upper part of the esophagus, aiding in processes like swallowing and vocalization.

THE VAGUS NERVE

Solitary Nucleus (Nucleus of the Solitary Tract):
- Location: The solitary nucleus is longitudinally elongated and is positioned laterally to the dorsal motor nucleus of the vagus nerve, medially by the medial eminence, and posteriorly by the area postrema. It extends from the level of the obex (the point in the medulla oblongata where the central canal of the spinal cord becomes the fourth ventricle) rostrally to the level of the area postrema.
- Function: This nucleus has both sensory and autonomic components. The sensory part processes taste sensations from the posterior third of the tongue and the outer ear. The autonomic component receives visceral sensory information (e.g., chemoreception and mechanoreception) from the thoracic and abdominal viscera.

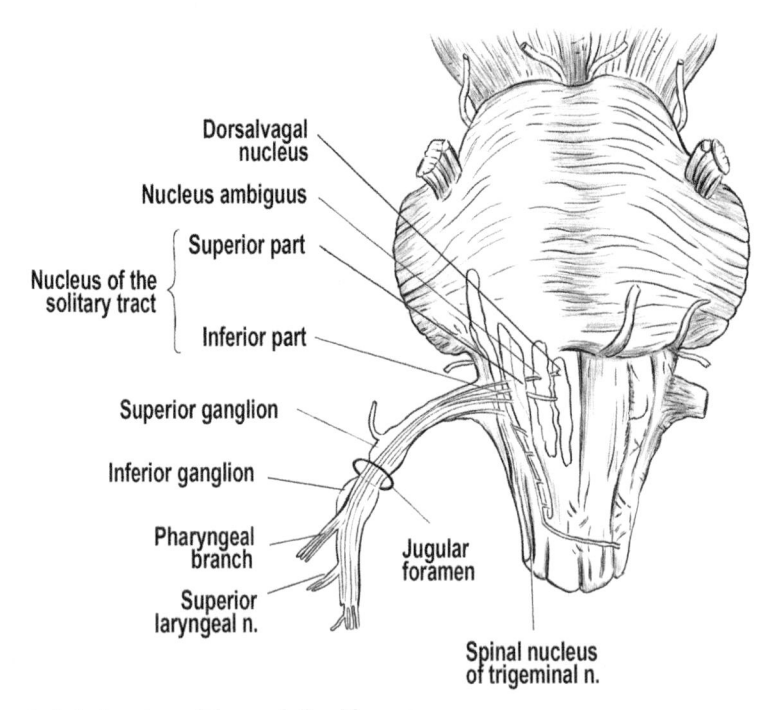

A Anterior view of the medulla oblongata.

[Diagram labels: Nucleus of the solitary tract (Superior part, Inferior part); Dorsal vagal nucleus; Spinal nucleus of trigeminal n.; Nucleus ambiguus; Olive]

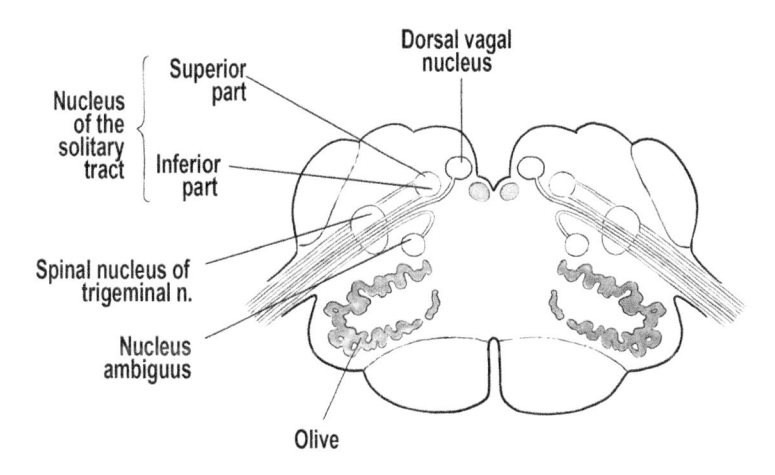

B Cross section through the medulla oblongata, superior view.

Spinal Trigeminal Nucleus:
- Location: The spinal trigeminal nucleus extends vertically through the medulla oblongata and descends into the cervical spinal cord, lying anterolaterally to the solitary nucleus in the medulla, and it stretches from the level of the pons down to the level of the cervical spinal cord.
- Function: Processes somatosensory information (e.g., pain, and temperature) from the outer ear, the dura of the posterior cranial fossa, and the mucosa of the larynx.

Anatomy: Ganglia

Superior Ganglion (Jugular Ganglion)
- Located in the jugular foramen. Contains the cell bodies of the afferent fibers from the meninges of the posterior cranial fossa and part of the external ear.

Inferior Ganglion (Nodose Ganglion)
- Situated just below the superior ganglion. Contains the cell bodies of

the afferent fibers from the pharynx, larynx, thoracic and abdominal viscera, and part of the external ear.

The Course of the Vagus Nerve

1. Exit from the Skull: The vagus nerve exits the skull through the jugular foramen, accompanied by the glossopharyngeal (CN IX) and accessory (CN XI) nerves and jugular vein.

2. Neck: After leaving the jugular foramen, the vagus nerve gives off the auricular branch which provides sensory innervation to a part of the external ear. As it descends in the neck, the vagus nerve travels within the carotid sheath, situated between the internal jugular vein and the common carotid artery. During its cervical course, it gives off several branches, including the pharyngeal branch (to the pharynx) and the superior laryngeal nerve (to the larynx).

3. Thorax: The vagus nerve enters the thorax and continues to give off branches to the heart, lungs, and esophagus. Two important branches in the thorax include the superior cardiac branches (to the heart) and the pulmonary branches (to the lungs). The nerve also provides fibers to the esophageal plexus, contributing to the motor control of the esophagus, facilitating peristalsis.

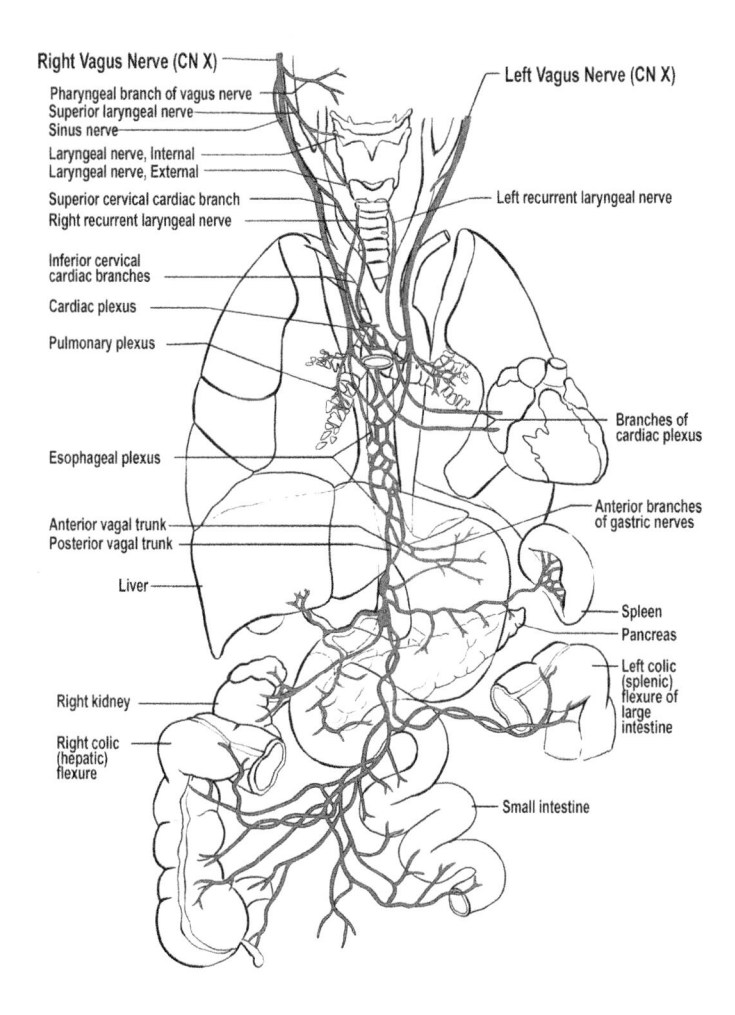

4. Abdomen: The vagus nerve enters the abdomen via the esophageal hiatus of the diaphragm. In the abdomen, it splits into the anterior and posterior vagal trunks. These trunks supply multiple abdominal organs, including the stomach, where they play a role in producing gastric secretions and controlling gastric motility. The vagus nerve's influence continues down through the intestines, reaching as far as the splenic flexure in the colon.

5. Termination: The vagal fibers spread out and terminate by synapsing with postganglionic neurons in various ganglia or directly on the smooth muscles and glands of the target organs.

The vagus nerve's extensive course and multifaceted innervation make it a key player in numerous physiological processes, especially within the parasympathetic division of the autonomic nervous system. It plays roles in the regulation of heart rate, gastrointestinal motility, respiratory rate, and more.

Important Vagal Pathways

Auricular Branch (Arnold's Nerve) of the Vagus Nerve:

The auricular branch arises from the inferior ganglion (nodose ganglion) of the vagus nerve. After branching off, it ascends to the ear by traveling alongside or within the wall of the internal jugular vein. It then penetrates the mastoid canaliculus, a tiny canal in the temporal bone, and makes its way into the temporal bone's mastoid air cells. Eventually, it reaches its target areas in the ear.

The auricular branch provides sensory innervation to the posterior and inferior parts of the external auditory canal's wall. This means that it's responsible for transmitting pain, temperature, touch, and pressure sensations from these regions.

Apart from the external auditory canal, Arnold's nerve also provides sensory innervation to the posterior-inferior quadrant of the tympanic membrane (eardrum). It's worth noting that the tympanic membrane is also innervated by other nerves like the glossopharyngeal nerve (Jacobson's nerve) and the trigeminal nerve (via the mandibular branch).

Finally, the auricular branch provides sensory innervation to the concha region and external auditory meatus of the ear as shown in the image. This is particularly important, as it is the primary area of electrical stimulation for non-invasive forms of vagus nerve stimulation. More on this later in the book.

THE VAGUS NERVE

Pharyngeal Branches of the Vagus Nerve:

The pharyngeal branches arise primarily from the inferior ganglion (nodose ganglion) of the vagus nerve. These branches collaborate with branches from the glossopharyngeal nerve (CN IX) to form the pharyngeal plexus, which is a network of nerve fibers supplying the pharynx's muscles and mucosa.

The vagus nerve provides sensory fibers to the mucosa of the lower part of the pharynx, especially the region around the laryngeal opening. It conveys sensations of touch, pain, temperature, and pressure from this region. These sensory fibers also play a role in initiating the swallowing reflex once food or liquid reaches the lower pharynx.

The vagus nerve, through its pharyngeal branches, innervates most of the muscles of the pharynx. This motor innervation is vital for the coordinated contractions required for the act of swallowing. Specifically, the muscles innervated by the vagus nerve include the superior, middle, and inferior constrictor muscles, which constrict the pharynx during swallowing, as well as the salpingopharyngeus and palatopharyngeus muscles, which help elevate the pharynx.

Clinical Significance:
- Dysphagia: Damage or dysfunction of the vagus nerve or its pharyngeal branches can lead to difficulty swallowing, known as dysphagia. This can result from various causes, including surgical trauma, tumors, or neurological disorders.
- Loss of Gag Reflex: The afferent (sensory) limb of the gag reflex is primarily mediated by the glossopharyngeal nerve (CN IX), which senses the irritative stimulus. The efferent (motor) limb, which leads to the actual gagging response, is mediated by the vagus nerve. Damage to either of these nerves can diminish or eliminate the gag reflex.

Superior Laryngeal Nerve (SLN):

The SLN branches off the vagus nerve high in the neck and then divides into the internal and external laryngeal nerves.

Internal Laryngeal Nerve:

It is primarily sensory. Provides sensory innervation to the laryngeal mucosa above the vocal cords.

External Laryngeal Nerve:

Supplies the cricothyroid muscle, which adjusts the tension of the vocal cords, thus modulating the pitch of the voice.

Recurrent Laryngeal Nerve (RLN):

The RLN branches from the vagus nerve in the thorax and then ascends to the larynx. Its pathway is unique because on the right side, it loops around the right subclavian artery, whereas on the left side, it loops around the arch of the aorta before ascending.

The RLN supplies all intrinsic muscles of the larynx except for the cricothyroid muscle. These muscles facilitate vocal cord movement, helping in voice production and airway protection.

Lastly, the RLN provides sensation to the laryngeal mucosa below the vocal cords.

Clinical Significance of Vagus Nerve Dysfunction:
- Vocal Cord Paralysis: Injury to the RLN can result in paralysis of the vocal cords. This can lead to hoarseness, voice changes, and even breathing difficulties in severe cases, especially if both sides are affected.
- Surgical Implications: The RLN is at risk during surgeries involving the thyroid gland, parathyroid glands, or anterior cervical spine. Its unique and somewhat tortuous path makes it vulnerable. Surgeons often take great care to identify and preserve this nerve during procedures.
- Aspiration: If the RLN is injured, it can lead to ineffective closure of the vocal cords. This can predispose individuals to aspiration, where food or liquids enter the trachea and potentially the lungs, which can lead to aspiration pneumonia.

- Change in Voice Pitch: Damage to the external branch of the SLN can lead to difficulty adjusting the pitch of the voice due to the cricothyroid muscle's role in modulating vocal cord tension.

References

1. Butt, M.F., Albusoda, A., Farmer, A.D. and Aziz, Q., 2020. 'The anatomical basis for transcutaneous auricular vagus nerve stimulation', Journal of Anatomy, 236(4), pp.588-611.

2. Cork, S.C., 2018. 'The role of the vagus nerve in appetite control: Implications for the pathogenesis of obesity', Journal of Neuroendocrinology, 30(11), e12643.

3. Gage, N.M. and Baars, B., 2018. Fundamentals of Cognitive Neuroscience: A Beginner's Guide. 2nd ed. Elsevier.

4. Komisaruk, B.R. and Frangos, E., 2022. 'Vagus nerve afferent stimulation: Projection into the brain, reflexive physiological, perceptual, and behavioral responses, and clinical relevance', Autonomic Neuroscience, 237, 102908.

5. Kuwabara, S., Goggins, E. and Tanaka, S., 2022. 'Neuroimmune Circuits Activated by Vagus Nerve Stimulation', Nephron, 146(3), pp.286-290.

6. Ottaviani, M.M. and Macefield, V.G., 2022. 'Structure and Functions of the Vagus Nerve in Mammals', Comprehensive Physiology, 12(4), pp.3989-4037.

7. Prescott, S.L. and Liberles, S.D., 2022. 'Internal senses of the vagus nerve', Neuron, 110(4), pp.579-599.

8. Purves, D., Augustine, G., Fitzpatrick, D., Hall, W., LaMantia, A., Mooney, R., Platt, M. and White, L. (eds.), 2017. Neuroscience: 6th Edition. Oxford University Press USA.

9. Squire, L., Berg, D., Bloom, F.E., du Lac, S., Ghosh, A. and Spitzer, N.C. (eds.), 2012. Fundamental Neuroscience. 4th ed. Elsevier.

Chapter 5
The Vagus Nerve and the Lungs

The vagus nerve, or cranial nerve X, is a pivotal nerve in the parasympathetic nervous system. Its role is extensive throughout the body, given that it provides parasympathetic innervation to many organs from the neck down to the third part of the transverse colon. In the context of the lungs, the vagus nerve has several key roles:

Bronchomotor Tone:
- The vagus nerve provides the primary parasympathetic innervation to the airways.
- Stimulation of the vagal fibers leads to bronchoconstriction, a constriction or narrowing of the bronchi and bronchioles. This reduces the amount of air entering the alveoli and is a mechanism that protects the lungs from potential harmful substances in the inhaled air.
- This response opposes the sympathetic nervous system's role in causing bronchodilation, which expands the airways.

Glandular Secretions:
- The vagus nerve stimulates the secretion of mucus in the bronchial tree. Mucus plays a vital role in trapping foreign particles and pathogens, facilitating their removal from the respiratory system.

Pulmonary Stretch Receptors:
- Located in the smooth muscle of the airways, these receptors detect the degree of lung inflation.
- When the lungs are inflated to a certain threshold, the stretch receptors are activated and send afferent signals via the vagus nerve

to the brain. This is known as the Hering-Breuer reflex. This reflex helps prevent over-inflation of the lungs. When the threshold is reached, it inhibits further inhalation, promoting exhalation and thereby regulating the depth and rate of breathing.

Pulmonary Irritant Receptors:
- These receptors are found between airway epithelial cells and are sensitive to noxious agents, like smoke, dust, or cold air.
- When activated, these receptors send signals through the vagus nerve, leading to reflex responses such as coughing, bronchoconstriction, and increased respiratory rate to expel or avoid the irritant.

Juxtacapillary (J) Receptors:
- Located near the capillaries in the alveolar septa, these receptors are sensitive to increased pulmonary capillary pressure.
- When activated, they send signals via the vagus nerve, leading to rapid, shallow breathing. This can be seen in conditions like pulmonary edema.

Pulmonary Vasculature:
- While the vagus nerve predominantly affects the lung airways, there's evidence to suggest it may also play a role in influencing the pulmonary vasculature, potentially leading to vasodilation.

Cough Reflex:
- Beyond the Hering-Breuer reflex, the vagus nerve is involved in various other reflexes, such as the cough reflex. Irritation of the airways, trachea, or bronchi can activate this reflex.

Clinical Implications of Vagus Nerve Dysfunction:
- Asthma: The vagus nerve helps regulate airway smooth muscle tone. Dysfunction in vagal tone might lead to irregular constriction of airway muscles, exacerbating asthma symptoms.
- Chronic Obstructive Pulmonary Disease (COPD): The vagus nerve influences bronchoconstriction and mucus secretion. Reduced vagal activity may contribute to airway inflammation and hyper-

responsiveness, worsening COPD symptoms.

- Sleep Apnea: The vagus nerve has a role in controlling involuntary muscle movements associated with breathing. Dysfunction could disrupt respiratory rhythm during sleep, potentially contributing to episodes of apnea.

- Bronchitis: The vagus nerve has anti-inflammatory effects that could influence bronchial inflammation. Vagal dysfunction could exacerbate the inflammatory response in bronchitis.

- Pneumonia: The vagus nerve's role in immune regulation may impact the body's response to lung infections. Inadequate vagal tone may contribute to impaired immune responses, affecting the course of pneumonia.

- Pulmonary Hypertension: Vagus nerve dysfunction could influence the release of vasoactive substances. Poor vagal regulation could contribute to irregular constriction of pulmonary vessels, exacerbating pulmonary hypertension.

- Pleuritis: The vagus nerve has anti-inflammatory properties. Dysfunction could exacerbate inflammation of the pleura, worsening pleuritis symptoms.

- Dyspnea (Shortness of Breath): Vagal influence on smooth muscle tone in the airways might cause feelings of breathlessness. Dysfunction in vagal tone may contribute to episodes of dyspnea by impacting airway responsiveness or sensation.

The vagus nerve, an integral part of the PNS, plays a multifaceted role in maintaining lung function and responding to various stimuli. From controlling bronchomotor tone to facilitating various reflex actions, its influence is deeply embedded in the pulmonary system. The clinical implications of its dysfunction are varied, encompassing a range of respiratory conditions. While it's clear that the vagus nerve plays a pivotal role in pulmonary health, it's equally important to recognize that respiratory conditions arise from a myriad of factors. Thus, understanding the vagus nerve's function provides just one piece of the intricate puzzle of pulmonary health. As always, deeper insights into any respiratory ailment and its etiology should be sought from healthcare professionals, ensuring a comprehensive and informed approach to treatment and care.

References

1. Antin-Ozerkis, D. E., Dela Cruz, C. S., Kotloff, R., Kotton, C. N., Grippi, M. and Pack, A. 2023. Fishman's Pulmonary Diseases and Disorders, 2-Volume Set, 6th ed. McGraw-Hill Education.

2. Burki, N. K. and Lee, L. Y. 2010. 'Mechanisms of dyspnea', Chest, 138(5), pp. 1196-201. doi: 10.1378/chest.10-0534.

3. Kollarik, M. and Undem, B. J. 2005. 'The role of vagal afferent nerves in chronic obstructive pulmonary disease', Proc Am Thorac Soc, 2(4), pp. 355-360; discussion 371-2. doi: 10.1513/pats.200504-033SR.

4. Luks, A. M. and West, J. B. 2020. West's Respiratory Physiology: The Essentials, 11th ed. Lippincott Williams & Wilkins, USA.

Chapter 6
The Vagus Nerve and the Heart

The heart, a vital organ that orchestrates the rhythm of life, operates under intricate systems of regulation. Central to these systems is the vagus nerve, a key player with profound influence on cardiac functions. This chapter delves into the multifaceted role of the vagus nerve in the heart, elucidating its significance and the potential implications of its dysfunction. Here are some of the key functions:

1. Cardiac Rate (Chronotropic Effect)
- The vagus nerve is primarily responsible for the parasympathetic control of the heart rate.
- When activated, it releases acetylcholine (ACh) onto the pacemaker cells of the sinoatrial (SA) node, which is the heart's primary pacemaker.
- ACh decreases the rate of spontaneous depolarization of these pacemaker cells, thereby slowing down the heart rate. This is known as a negative chronotropic effect.
- Conversely, when there's reduced vagal tone compared to sympathetic activity, the heart rate increases.

2. Cardiac Conduction (Dromotropic Effect)
- The vagus nerve can influence the conduction velocity of electrical impulses in the heart, particularly at the atrioventricular (AV) node.
- By releasing ACh, the vagus nerve increases the refractory period of the AV node, slowing down the conduction of impulses from the atria to the ventricles. This is called a negative dromotropic effect.

3. Cardiac Contractility (Inotropic Effect)

- While the sympathetic nervous system has a pronounced influence on the contractility of the heart's chambers, the parasympathetic system, via the vagus nerve, has a lesser effect.
- Nevertheless, there's some evidence to suggest that intense parasympathetic stimulation can slightly reduce the force of the heart's contraction (negative inotropic effect), especially in the atria.

4. Reflex Control (Baroreflex)

- The vagus nerve is involved in the baroreflex, a critical reflex in the regulation of blood pressure.
- When high-pressure baroreceptors (found in the aortic arch and carotid sinus) detect an increase in blood pressure, they send signals via sensory fibers. These signals eventually result in increased parasympathetic activity via the vagus nerve and reduced sympathetic activity.
- This leads to a reduction in heart rate and, to a lesser extent, reduced cardiac contractility, causing a drop in blood pressure.

5. Protection against Cardiac Injury

- Recent research suggests that vagal stimulation can have a protective effect against cardiac injury, particularly ischemic injury (damage caused by reduced blood flow).
- This may be due to multiple factors, including anti-inflammatory effects, modulation of the immune response, and direct actions on cardiac cells.

6. Influence on Cardiac Arrhythmias

- The vagus nerve can have both pro-arrhythmic and anti-arrhythmic effects.
- For instance, excessive vagal tone can sometimes lead to a type of bradycardia (slow heart rate) called sinus bradycardia or to AV block (a delay or block in conduction from the atria to the ventricles).
- On the other hand, vagal stimulation has been proposed as a potential

treatment for certain types of tachyarrhythmias (fast rhythms).

Clinical Implications of Vagus Nerve Dysfunction:
- Arrhythmia: Dysfunction in the vagus nerve can lead to irregular heartbeats or arrhythmias, as the nerve is responsible for maintaining a steady heart rate. Imbalanced vagal activity can disrupt the heart's natural rhythm.
- Tachycardia: When the vagus nerve is underactive, it may result in an elevated heart rate, known as tachycardia. The nerve's role in slowing down the heart rate is compromised, causing rapid beats.
- Bradycardia: Overactive vagal tone can cause the heart rate to slow down excessively, leading to bradycardia. In extreme cases, this can result in fainting or cardiac arrest.
- Heart Failure: In heart failure, an impaired vagus nerve may contribute to worsened cardiac function. Some studies suggest vagus nerve stimulation may improve outcomes by helping to regulate heart rate and contraction strength.
- Hypertension: Vagal nerve dysfunction can impact the body's ability to regulate blood pressure, potentially leading to hypertension or worsening existing high blood pressure.
- Atrial Fibrillation: Abnormal vagal activity can destabilize the electrical impulses in the heart, contributing to atrial fibrillation, a common and often serious arrhythmia.
- Postural Orthostatic Tachycardia Syndrome (POTS): Dysfunctional vagal tone may exacerbate symptoms of POTS, such as an abnormal increase in heart rate upon standing up.
- Sudden Cardiac Arrest: Low vagal tone has been linked to a higher risk for sudden cardiac arrest. A dysfunctional vagus nerve may fail to regulate heart rate effectively during stress, contributing to the risk.
- Myocardial Infarction (Heart Attack): Reduced vagal activity can worsen the outcome after a heart attack by failing to modulate inflammatory responses, thereby increasing the area of heart muscle

damage.

- Endothelial Dysfunction: The vagus nerve plays a role in regulating endothelial cells that line blood vessels. Dysfunction can lead to reduced vasodilation, contributing to cardiovascular diseases.

- Peripheral Artery Disease (PAD): Dysfunction in the vagus nerve could potentially impair blood flow to extremities, exacerbating symptoms of PAD like leg pain or numbness.

- Stroke: A dysfunctional vagus nerve may compromise any neuroprotective effects it might offer during a stroke, possibly affecting recovery and long-term outcomes.

The intricate relationship between the vagus nerve and the heart underscores the importance of the PNS in cardiac function. Through its multifarious roles, ranging from influencing the heart rate to potential protection against cardiac injury, the vagus nerve stands out as a critical regulator of cardiovascular health. Aberrations in its function can manifest in various cardiovascular diseases, making it a potential therapeutic target in cardiology. However, it's imperative to remember that while the vagus nerve plays a pivotal role in heart health, it's only one part of the complex system that governs cardiovascular function. A holistic understanding, encompassing all potential etiologies, is essential for optimal patient care. As with all medical concerns, collaboration with healthcare professionals ensures informed decisions and evidence-based treatments.

References

1. Atkinson, L., Deuchars, J., Deuchars, S. A., Mahadi, M. K. and Murray, A. R. 2016. 'The strange case of the ear and the heart: The auricular vagus nerve and its influence on cardiac control', Auton Neurosci, 199, pp. 48-53. doi: 10.1016/j.autneu.2016.06.004.

2. Becker, L. B., Capilupi, M. J. and Kerath, S. M. 2020. 'Vagus Nerve Stimulation and the Cardiovascular System', Cold Spring Harb Perspect Med, 10(2), a034173. doi: 10.1101/cshperspect.a034173.

3. Bender, S. A., Daniels, R. J., Ganoadra, N., Green, D. B. and Vrabec, T. L. 2023. 'Effects on heart rate from direct current block of the stimulated rat vagus nerve', J Neural Eng, 20(1). doi: 10.1088/1741-2552/acacc9.

4. Frullini, S., Haberbusch, M. and Moscato, F. 2022. 'A Numerical Model of the Acute Cardiac Effects Provoked by Cervical Vagus Nerve Stimulation', IEEE Trans Biomed Eng, 69(2), pp. 613-623. doi: 10.1109/TBME.2021.3102416.

5. Holler, T. 2007. Cardiology Essentials, 1st ed. Jones and Bartlett Publishers, Inc. ISBN: 9780763750763.

6. Jiang, H., Po, S. S., Scherlag, B. J., Wang, Y. and Yu, L. 2019. 'The role of low-level vagus nerve stimulation in cardiac therapy', Expert Rev Med Devices, 16(8), pp. 675-682. doi: 10.1080/17434440.2019.1643234.

7. Kronsteiner, B., Aigner, P., Haberbusch, M., Kiss, A., Kramer, A. M., Moscato, F. and Podesser, B. K. 2023. 'A novel ex-vivo isolated rabbit heart preparation to explore the cardiac effects of cervical and cardiac vagus nerve stimulation', Sci Rep, 13(1), 4214. doi: 10.1038/s41598-023-31135-4.

Chapter 7
The Vagus Nerve and Swallowing

Swallowing is a multi-step, highly coordinated physiological process that allows us to consume food and liquids safely. While multiple nerves and muscles are involved in this complex mechanism, the vagus nerve (Cranial Nerve X) plays a critical role in its orchestration. This chapter aims to provide a comprehensive overview of the relationship between the vagus nerve and the act of swallowing, addressing the underlying anatomy, functional implications, and clinical ramifications.

Origin and Pathway:

The vagus nerve follows a long descending path from the medulla oblongata through to the neck, within the carotid sheath, sharing space with key arteries and veins. Once it reaches the pharynx, it branches out to innervate the various structures involved in swallowing.

Pharyngeal Plexus:

The pharyngeal plexus is a network of intertwined nerves from the vagus, glossopharyngeal, and sympathetic nerves. This plexus provides the innervation essential for the sensory and motor functions of the pharynx, facilitating complex actions like swallowing and speech.

Target Muscles:

The superior, middle, and inferior pharyngeal constrictor muscles receive innervation from the vagus nerve. These muscles work in concert to narrow the pharynx during swallowing, pushing food toward the esophagus.

Sensory and Motor Fibers:

The vagus nerve contains both sensory and motor fibers, a feature that serves a dual purpose. Sensory fibers collect information on stretch and tension within the pharyngeal muscles, which informs swallowing reflexes. Motor fibers relay commands for muscle contraction and relaxation.

Processes Involved in Swallowing:

Oral Preparatory Phase

1. Buccal Tension Reflex

   - Description: The buccal tension reflex is triggered when food is placed in the mouth. Sensory neurons in the cheeks send signals to the brainstem, which in turn commands muscles to contract and maintain food within the oral cavity.
   - Role of Vagus Nerve: Although primarily managed by facial and trigeminal nerves, the vagus nerve's sensory fibers can help modulate this reflex, particularly if the food bolus reaches the back of the oral cavity.

Oral Phase

2. Tongue-Palate Reflex

   - Description: The tongue moves food against the hard palate to form a bolus, a process triggered by sensory feedback.
   - Role of Vagus Nerve: The vagus nerve is minimally involved here but contributes to the general coordination of the swallowing reflexes.

Pharyngeal Phase

3. Gag Reflex

   - Description: Triggered by the touching of the posterior pharyngeal wall, this reflex initiates a strong contraction of the pharyngeal muscles to prevent choking.
   - Role of Vagus Nerve: The vagus nerve's sensory fibers play a crucial role in detecting stimuli that trigger the gag reflex, and its motor

fibers help execute it.

4. Upper Esophageal Sphincter (UES) Opening
   - Description: The UES relaxes to allow the passage of the food bolus into the esophagus.
   - Role of Vagus Nerve: The vagus nerve commands the relaxation of the cricopharyngeus muscle, which composes part of the UES.

Esophageal Phase

5. Peristaltic Reflex
   - Description: Sequential muscle contractions move the food bolus down the esophagus.
   - Role of Vagus Nerve: The vagus nerve coordinates these muscular contractions, ensuring effective peristalsis.

6. Lower Esophageal Sphincter (LES) Opening
   - Description: The LES relaxes to allow the food bolus to enter the stomach.
   - Role of Vagus Nerve: Parasympathetic fibers of the vagus nerve command the relaxation of the LES.

Additional Reflexes

7. Respiratory Pause Reflex
   - Description: Swallowing briefly inhibits respiration to prevent aspiration.
   - Role of Vagus Nerve: The vagus nerve communicates with the respiratory centers in the medulla to coordinate this brief cessation of breathing.

8. Cough Reflex
   - Description: If aspiration is detected, a cough reflex is triggered to expel foreign material from the airway.
   - Role of Vagus Nerve: The vagus nerve's sensory fibers detect the

aspirated material and its motor fibers help in initiating the cough reflex.

Each of these reflexes involves intricate neural pathways that ensure the smooth, coordinated action of swallowing. Understanding their description is essential for the diagnosis and treatment of swallowing disorders.

Clinical Implications of Vagus Nerve Dysfunction:

Swallowing Disorders: An impaired vagus nerve can lead to dysphagia or difficulty in swallowing. Since the vagus nerve plays a role in coordinating the muscles involved in the swallowing process and provides secretomotor function to the minor salivary and mucous glands, any disruption can lead to reduced lubrication and coordination, making swallowing challenging.

References

1. Costa, M.M.B. 2018. 'NEURAL CONTROL OF SWALLOWING', Arq Gastroenterol, 55(Suppl 1), pp. 61-75. doi: 10.1590/S0004-2803.201800000-45.

2. Jean, A. 2001. 'Brain stem control of swallowing: neuronal network and cellular mechanisms', Physiol Rev, 81(2), pp. 929-969. doi: 10.1152/physrev.2001.81.2.929.

3. Pitts, T. 2014. 'Airway protective mechanisms', Lung, 192(1), pp. 27-31. doi: 10.1007/s00408-013-9540-y.

4. Prescott, S. L., Brust, R. D., Liberles, S. D., Umans, B. D. and Williams, E. K. 2020. 'An Airway Protection Program Revealed by Sweeping Genetic Control of Vagal Afferents', Cell, 181(3), pp. 574-589.e14. doi: 10.1016/j.cell.2020.03.004.

Chapter 8
The Vagus Nerve and Speech

The ability to produce speech is one of the most distinctive features of human communication, setting us apart from other species. Speech is a symphony of coordinated neural activities that span different regions of the brain, various cranial nerves, and a plethora of muscles. Among these, the vagus nerve emerges as a seminal conductor in the orchestration, playing an instrumental role in the nuanced activities needed for speech production. Its involvement is not just isolated to one facet of speech but extends across the continuum of voice production, modulation, and resonance. Understanding the role of the vagus nerve in speech is not merely academic; it holds clinical significance for diagnosing and treating speech disorders, aiding in surgical planning, and even has implications in the fields of psychology and social interaction.

The vagus nerve, emerging from the medulla oblongata, follows a trajectory from the brainstem, exits the skull via the jugular foramen, and descends through the neck within the carotid sheath. Along its path, it branches to serve various physiological roles. A significant branch for speech is the recurrent laryngeal nerve, which innervates many of the larynx's intrinsic muscles. This nerve notably loops under the right subclavian artery and the aortic arch on the left, before rerouting to the larynx - a feature with clinical relevance, especially when surrounding arteries are involved in surgical or pathological scenarios.

The vagus nerve's motor fibers are instrumental in voice modulation by adjusting the vocal cords' position, tension, and length. Meanwhile, its sensory fibers provide feedback from the larynx and nearby structures, aiding in reflexive speech adjustments. To fine-tune speech, the vagus nerve collaborates with previously mentioned nerves and various regions, ensuring a coordinated effort for optimal articulation and voice production. Now we will consider all the physiological processes involved:

Phonation

Phonation refers to the process of producing sound by the vibration of the vocal folds within the larynx, which is modulated by the airflow from the lungs.

Vocal Fold Adduction and Abduction: Phonation begins with the adduction of the vocal folds, essentially bringing them close enough to touch or almost touch each other. The motor fibers of the recurrent laryngeal nerve stimulate the intrinsic muscles of the larynx, such as the thyroarytenoid and lateral cricoarytenoid muscles, to facilitate this action. Conversely, abduction of the vocal folds occurs when these fibers stimulate the posterior cricoarytenoid muscles, opening the vocal folds to allow for respiration. The fine-tuned control of adduction and abduction is vital for seamless transition between speech and breathing.

Voice Pitch and Intensity: Pitch and intensity of the voice are determined by how tightly the vocal folds are stretched and how fast they vibrate. The cricothyroid muscle, controlled by the recurrent laryngeal nerve, adjusts the tension by tilting the thyroid cartilage. This modulation impacts the pitch. Voice intensity is altered by changing subglottal pressure, which is regulated by respiratory muscles but coordinated through vagal nerve activity.

Vocal Fold Sensory Feedback: Sensory fibers within the vagus nerve gather information from the laryngeal mucosa and vocal folds. This feedback helps in making real-time adjustments during speech, such as correcting pitch or avoiding voice breaks.

Resonance and Timbre

Resonance: The amplification and enrichment of voice sounds as they pass through the cavities of the throat, mouth, and nose, shaping the overall quality and character of the voice. The vagus nerve plays a part in shaping these contours by controlling some muscles of the soft palate, indirectly affecting the resonance characteristics of speech.

Timbre: Timbre refers to the unique quality or color of a voice that distinguishes it from others. While the vagus nerve is not solely responsible for timbre, it plays a part by influencing the vibrational characteristics of the vocal folds and modulating the shape of the vocal tract.

Articulation

Articulation refers to the movement and coordination of the tongue, lips, palate, and other oral structures to produce clear and distinct speech sounds.

Role in Tongue and Palate Movement: While the primary muscles involved in articulation (like tongue muscles) are controlled by other cranial nerves such as the hypoglossal nerve, the vagus nerve does contribute to some extent. For instance, it innervates the palatoglossus muscle, which draws the back of the tongue upward. This action is important in creating specific speech sounds and in separating the oral and nasal cavities during speech and swallowing.

Coordinated Activity: Articulation involves the complex interplay between various muscles and neural inputs. The vagus nerve works in concert with other cranial nerves and cortical areas to synchronize movements like lip rounding, tongue elevation, and palate lifting, which are crucial for the distinct articulation of phonemes.

By understanding these complex mechanisms of phonation, resonance, timbre, and articulation, and the role the vagus nerve plays in each, clinicians and speech therapists can better diagnose and treat speech disorders. Moreover, the information lays the groundwork for potential interventions like targeted vagus nerve stimulation to improve speech outcomes.

Clinical Implications of Vagus Nerve Dysfunction:
- Vocal Fold Paralysis or Paresis: This condition involves the loss or reduction of function in the vocal folds, making it difficult to speak, breathe, or swallow. Damage to the recurrent laryngeal nerve, a

branch of the vagus nerve, can lead to vocal fold paralysis or paresis, affecting voice quality and respiratory function.

- Dysphonia: Dysphonia refers to disorders of the voice, which may manifest as hoarseness, breathiness, or reduced pitch or volume. Irregular signaling from the vagus nerve to the laryngeal muscles can disrupt the mechanics of voice production, leading to various forms of dysphonia.

- Spasmodic Dysphonia: This is a neurological voice disorder characterized by involuntary spasms in the muscles of the larynx, affecting speech quality. Malfunctioning vagus nerve signaling can cause abnormal contractions in the laryngeal muscles, resulting in the characteristic spasms of spasmodic dysphonia.

- Speech Resonance Disorders: These include hypernasality and hyponasality, conditions where speech sounds excessively nasal or lacks normal nasal resonance. Impaired vagus nerve function can affect the muscles that control the palate, leading to poor separation of oral and nasal cavities during speech, causing resonance issues.

- Aphonia: Aphonia refers to the complete loss of voice where the person can only whisper. Severe dysfunction or damage to the vagus nerve can result in the complete inability to adduct the vocal folds, leading to aphonia.

In sum, the multifaceted role of the vagus nerve in speech production, modulation, and resonance is paramount to our understanding of human communication. Its intricate pathways and nuanced functions underscore the complexity of our vocal mechanisms, from the delicate dance of vocal folds during phonation to the subtle intricacies in articulation. Recognizing its significance extends beyond academic appreciation—it's crucial for clinicians, surgeons, and therapists aiming to diagnose and rectify speech disorders. As we delve deeper into the intricacies of the vagus nerve, we pave the way for advanced therapeutic interventions, offering a beacon of hope for those grappling with communication challenges.

References

1. Duffy, J.R. 2019. Motor Speech Disorders: Substrates, Differential Diagnosis, and Management, 4th ed. Elsevier US.

2. Laccourreye, O., Malinvaud, D., Ménard, M. and Bonfils, P. 2014. 'Paralysies laryngées unilatérales de l'adulte: épidémiologie, symptomatologie, physiopathologie et traitement', Presse Med, 43(4 Pt 1), pp. 348-352. doi: 10.1016/j.lpm.2013.07.029.

3. Ludlow, C.L., Adler, C.H., Berke, G.S., Bielamowicz, S.A., Blitzer, A., Bressman, S.B., Hallett, M., Jinnah, H.A., Juergens, U., Martin, S.B., Perlmutter, J.S., Sapienza, C., Singleton, A., Tanner, C.M. and Woodson, G.E. 2008. 'Research priorities in spasmodic dysphonia', Otolaryngol Head Neck Surg, 139(4), pp. 495-505. doi: 10.1016/j.otohns.2008.05.624.

4. Miyauchi, A., Inoue, H., Tomoda, C., Fukushima, M., Kihara, M., Higashiyama, T., Takamura, Y., Ito, Y., Kobayashi, K. and Miya, A. 2009. 'Improvement in phonation after reconstruction of the recurrent laryngeal nerve in patients with thyroid cancer invading the nerve', Surgery, 146(6), pp. 1056-1062. doi: 10.1016/j.surg.2009.09.018.

5. Morrison, R.A., Hays, S.A. and Kilgard, M.P. 2021. 'Vagus Nerve Stimulation as a Potential Adjuvant to Rehabilitation for Post-stroke Motor Speech Disorders', Front Neurosci, 15, 715928. doi: 10.3389/fnins.2021.715928.

6. Salik, I. and Winters, R. 2023. 'Bilateral Vocal Cord Paralysis'. In: StatPearls [Internet]. Treasure Island (FL): StatPearls Publishing; 2023 Jan–.

Chapter 9
The Vagus Nerve and the Esophagus

The vagus nerve (cranial nerve X) has an integral role in the function of the esophagus, which is a muscular tube that connects the pharynx (throat) to the stomach. It is responsible for transporting food and liquids from the mouth to the stomach through coordinated muscular contractions known as peristalsis. Here's how the vagus nerve is involved:

Esophageal Branches of the Vagus Nerve:

Both the left and right vagus nerves give off anterior and posterior esophageal branches. These branches contribute to the formation of the esophageal plexus, a complex network of nerve fibers surrounding the esophagus. These fibers innervate the muscular layers of the esophagus. The upper third of the esophagus consists of striated (voluntary) muscle, and its peristaltic contractions are primarily controlled by the vagus. The lower two-thirds of the esophagus is smooth (involuntary) muscle. Here, the vagus nerve helps coordinate the peristaltic waves that propel food toward the stomach.

The vagus nerve also supplies sensory fibers to the esophagus. These fibers help detect stretching and other mechanical changes, providing feedback that influences motor responses. The nerve plays a role in initiating the primary peristaltic wave upon swallowing and helps mediate secondary peristaltic waves when any residue is detected.

Lower Esophageal Sphincter (LES):

The LES is a muscular ring at the lower end of the esophagus, just before it enters the stomach. The vagus nerve helps regulate the tone of the LES. When food approaches, the LES relaxes, allowing it to enter the stomach.

Afterward, the LES contracts again to prevent reflux of stomach contents back into the esophagus.

Clinical Significance of Vagus Nerve Dysfunction:

- Dysphagia: The vagus nerve plays a direct role in the coordination of swallowing. Any disruption in its function can impede this coordination, resulting in dysphagia. This swallowing difficulty can emerge from neuromuscular disorders, direct compression of the vagus nerve, or complications post-surgery where the nerve might be affected.

- Gastroesophageal Reflux Disease (GERD): The LES's tonality, which the vagus nerve directly regulates, is essential for preventing stomach acid backflow. Vagal dysfunction can lead to an abnormal relaxation of the LES, causing acid reflux into the esophagus. GERD symptoms include heartburn and regurgitation, and prolonged exposure can lead to more severe complications, such as esophagitis.

- Achalasia: In achalasia, the LES doesn't relax as it should, resulting in food being trapped in the lower esophagus. The vagus nerve indirectly influences this condition through its role in the myenteric plexus, where a loss of inhibitory neurons can lead to the LES's malfunction.

- Barrett's Esophagus: While the vagus nerve doesn't directly cause Barrett's esophagus, its potential role in the genesis or exacerbation of GERD can indirectly contribute to this condition. Chronic GERD, potentially influenced by vagal dysfunction affecting LES tonality, can lead to changes in the esophageal lining, culminating in Barrett's esophagus. This condition requires continuous monitoring due to the increased risk of esophageal cancer.

The intricate relationship between the vagus nerve and the esophagus is paramount to the seamless process of swallowing and digestion. As the esophagus serves as a conduit for food, the vagus nerve orchestrates its muscular activities, ensuring the smooth transition of food from the mouth to the stomach. Moreover, any dysfunction of this nerve can manifest in a spectrum of esophageal disorders, underscoring the importance of understanding its anatomy and physiology. This knowledge is essential not only for grasping basic human biology but also for the diagnosis and treatment of various esophageal conditions. As we delve deeper into the complexities of the human body, the indispensable role of the vagus nerve in esophageal function stands out as a testament to the body's intricate design and coordination.

References

1. Brock, C., Brokjaer, A., Drewes, A.M., Farmer, A.D., Frøkjaer, J.B., Gregersen, H. and Lottrup, C. 2014. 'Neurophysiology of the esophagus', Ann N Y Acad Sci, 1325, pp. 57-68. doi: 10.1111/nyas.12515.

2. Jean, A. 2001. 'Brain stem control of swallowing: neuronal network and cellular mechanisms', Physiol Rev, 81(2), pp. 929-969. doi: 10.1152/physrev.2001.81.2.929.

3. Neuhuber, W.L., Raab, M., Berthoud, H.R. and Wörl, J. 2006. 'Innervation of the mammalian esophagus', Adv Anat Embryol Cell Biol, 185, pp. 1-73.

4. Wörl, J. and Neuhuber, W.L. 2005. 'Enteric co-innervation of motor endplates in the esophagus: state of the art ten years after', Histochem Cell Biol, 123(2), pp. 117-130. doi: 10.1007/s00418-005-0764-7.

Chapter 10
The Vagus Nerve and the Stomach

The vagus nerve (cranial nerve X) has a profound influence on the stomach. Its involvement is crucial for several aspects of gastric physiology, especially given its role in the parasympathetic nervous system. Here's an in-depth analysis of the vagus nerve's role in stomach function:

1. Gastric Motility:

- Stomach Contractions: The vagus nerve influences the rhythmic contractions of the stomach muscles, ensuring efficient churning and mixing of food with gastric secretions to form chyme.

- Gastric Emptying: The vagus nerve helps regulate the rate at which the stomach empties its contents into the duodenum of the small intestine.

- Coordination with Pyloric Sphincter: The vagus nerve helps in coordinating the relaxation of the pyloric sphincter. This relaxation is essential for the chyme to move from the stomach to the duodenum.

2. Gastric Secretion:

- Acid Production: The vagus nerve stimulates parietal cells in the stomach lining to produce hydrochloric acid. This acid is essential for digestion, particularly for the breakdown of proteins.

- Enzyme Production: The nerve also stimulates chief cells to secrete pepsinogen, a precursor to the enzyme pepsin, which also plays a role in protein digestion.

- Hormonal Influence: The vagus nerve stimulates the release of gastrin, a hormone that promotes acid secretion and gastric motility.

3. Gastroprotective Role:
- The vagus nerve stimulates the secretion of mucus by mucous cells in the stomach. This mucus forms a protective barrier that shields the stomach lining from the corrosive effects of hydrochloric acid.

4. Gastric Reflexes:
- Vagovagal Reflex: This reflex involves both afferent and efferent fibers of the vagus nerve. For instance, distension of the stomach (when it fills with food) can trigger a reflexive increase in gastric secretions and motility.
- Gastrocolic Reflex: Following food ingestion and gastric distension, there's an increase in colonic motility. While this reflex involves multiple pathways, the vagus nerve plays a role in its initiation.

5. Sensory Functions:
- The vagus nerve conveys sensory information from the stomach to the brain. This includes sensations of fullness, discomfort, or pain.
- It also senses chemical changes within the stomach, like changes in pH, which can influence gastric secretion and motility reflexes.

6. Hunger and Satiety:
- While the exact mechanisms are complex and multifaceted, the vagus nerve is involved in transmitting signals related to hunger and satiety. This communication is partly based on the stretch of the stomach (indicating fullness) and chemical signals from the gastrointestinal tract and hormones.

7. Protection against Damage:
- Ischemic or other types of damage to the stomach lining can be counteracted by vagal stimulation. This protective effect might be due to increased mucus and bicarbonate secretion, enhanced blood flow, and other anti-inflammatory and cytoprotective mechanisms.

THE VAGUS NERVE AND THE STOMACH

Clinical Implications of Vagus Nerve Dysfunction:

- Gastroparesis: This condition, characterized by delayed gastric emptying in the absence of any mechanical obstruction, can arise due to impaired vagus nerve function. The stomach's muscles don't contract properly, leading to symptoms like nausea, vomiting, and bloating.

- Functional Dyspepsia: Though the exact cause of functional dyspepsia isn't clear, altered vagal activity may contribute to the stomach discomfort, bloating, and pain seen in this condition.

- Postoperative Nausea and Vomiting (PONV): Surgeries, especially those involving the upper abdomen, can impact the vagus nerve, leading to gastric stasis and the potential for nausea and vomiting postoperatively.

- Dumping Syndrome: Often a complication after gastric surgeries like gastric bypass or partial gastrectomy, this syndrome is characterized by rapid gastric emptying. Cutting the vagus nerve during surgery can lead to this condition, resulting in symptoms like nausea, vomiting, abdominal cramps, and dizziness.

- Bezoars: These are solid masses made up of food or hair that can be found in the stomach. They can form as a result of gastroparesis or impaired gastric motility due to vagus nerve dysfunction.

- Bariatric Surgery Complications: Certain bariatric surgeries can affect the vagus nerve either directly or indirectly, leading to alterations in gastric motility or acid secretion.

The vagus nerve stands as a central figure in the stomach's physiology, orchestrating a myriad of functions from gastric motility and secretion to intricate feedback mechanisms related to hunger and fullness. Its dual role as a sensory and motor nerve ensures a seamless bidirectional communication between the stomach and the central nervous system. Beyond its physiological duties, the nerve's dysfunctions underscore its significance, as evident in conditions like gastroparesis, functional dyspepsia, and postoperative complications. As we delve deeper into understanding the multifaceted interactions between the vagus nerve and the stomach, the knowledge paves the way for improved treatment strategies and a comprehensive approach to digestive health.

References

1. Powley, T.L., Jaffey, D.M., McAdams, J., Baronowsky, E.A., Black, D., Chesney, L., Evans, C. and Phillips, R.J., 2019. 'Vagal innervation of the stomach reassessed: brain-gut connectome uses smart terminals', Ann N Y Acad Sci, 1454(1), pp.14-30. doi: 10.1111/nyas.14138.

2. Schemann, M., Rohn, M. and Michel, K., 2008. 'Motor control of the stomach', Eur Rev Med Pharmacol Sci, 12 Suppl 1, pp.41-51. PMID: 18924443.

3. Skandalakis, J.E., Gray, S.W., Soria, R.E., Sorg, J.L. and Rowe, J.S. Jr., 1980. 'Distribution of the vagus nerve to the stomach', Am Surg, 46(3), pp.130-139. PMID: 7377655.

4. Steidel, K., Krause, K., Menzler, K., Strzelczyk, A., Immisch, I., Fuest, S., Gorny, I., Mross, P., Hakel, L., Schmidt, L., Timmermann, L., Rosenow, F., Bauer, S. and Knake, S., 2021. 'Transcutaneous auricular vagus nerve stimulation influences gastric motility: A randomized, double-blind trial in healthy individuals', Brain Stimul, 14(5), pp.1126-1132. doi: 10.1016/j.brs.2021.06.006.

5. Tao, J., Campbell, J.N., Tsai, L.T., Wu, C., Liberles, S.D. and Lowell, B.B., 2021. 'Highly selective brain-to-gut communication via genetically defined vagus neurons', Neuron, 109(13), pp.2106-2115.e4. doi: 10.1016/j.neuron.2021.05.004.

Chapter 11
The Vagus Nerve and the Small Intestines

The vagus nerve plays a significant role in the physiology and functioning of the small intestines. The nerve has both sensory (afferent) and motor (efferent) fibers that help in various aspects of digestion, absorption, and gut-brain communication.

1. Motility:

- Peristalsis: The vagus nerve influences the rhythmic contractions that propel chyme (partially digested food) through the small intestines, a process known as peristalsis.

- Segmentation: This is a coordinated local contraction that aids in mixing chyme with digestive enzymes and ensuring contact with the absorptive surfaces of the intestines. The vagus nerve contributes to the regulation of this process.

2. Secretion:

- Enteric Peptides and Hormones: The vagus nerve modulates the release of various peptides and hormones in the small intestine, which can influence digestion, absorption, and even appetite.

- Pancreatic Enzyme Secretion: While direct control of pancreatic secretion comes from hormones like cholecystokinin (CCK) and secretin released in the small intestine, the vagus nerve does play an indirect and modulatory role. Pancreatic enzymes are essential for the digestion of fats, proteins, and carbohydrates.

3. Absorption:

- While the vagus nerve doesn't directly control absorption, the efficient mixing of chyme and its movement against the intestines' absorptive walls, facilitated by the vagus nerve, is vital for optimal nutrient uptake.

4. Gut-Brain Communication:

- Nutrient Sensing: The vagus nerve's receptors can detect various nutrients in the intestine, relaying this information to the brain, influencing feelings of satiety and energy homeostasis.

- Gut-Brain Axis: The vagus nerve is a critical component of the gut-brain axis, allowing for bidirectional communication between the gastrointestinal tract and the central nervous system. This pathway plays a role in appetite regulation, mood, and overall gut function.

5. Protection and Repair:

- Mucosal Blood Flow: Vagal stimulation can influence blood flow to the mucosal lining of the intestines, which can promote healing and repair after injury.

- Immune Regulation: The vagus nerve can modulate immune responses in the intestines, playing a role in the balance between inflammation and tolerance.

6. Ileogastric Reflex:

- The vagus nerve is pivotal in mediating the ileogastric reflex, which inhibits stomach motility and secretions if the ileum, the last segment of the small intestines, becomes distended. This prevention ensures no overload of chyme in the small intestine.

7. Enteric Nervous System Interaction:

- The small intestine possesses its own intrinsic nervous system: the enteric nervous system (ENS). Although the ENS operates autonomously, the vagus nerve offers modulatory feedback, harmonizing central and local intestinal control.

Clinical Significance of Vagus Nerve Dysfunction:
- Gastrointestinal Motility Disorders: The vagus nerve is essential for the rhythmic contractions of the small intestine known as peristalsis. Dysfunction can lead to erratic or absent peristaltic activity. Reduced signaling from the vagus nerve can disrupt the natural motility of the intestine, leading to conditions like ileus or chronic intestinal pseudo-obstruction.
- Small Intestinal Bacterial Overgrowth (SIBO): Altered motility due to vagus nerve dysfunction can result in bacterial overgrowth in the small intestine. When the natural flow of contents through the small intestine is disrupted, it creates an environment where bacteria can proliferate.
- Postoperative Ileus: Sometimes, surgeries involving the abdominal area can impact the vagus nerve or its signaling. This disruption can inhibit intestinal motility, contributing to postoperative ileus, where the intestine temporarily stops functioning.
- Dumping Syndrome: Vagus nerve dysfunction can lead to rapid emptying of stomach contents into the small intestine. The vagus nerve usually helps regulate the pyloric sphincter, and its dysfunction can cause the sphincter to open prematurely, leading to dumping syndrome.
- Malabsorption Syndromes: Altered vagus nerve function can affect intestinal secretion and motility. Disruption in these processes can result in inefficient nutrient absorption, leading to various malabsorption syndromes like steatorrhea.
- Irritable Bowel Syndrome (IBS): While not directly a vagus nerve disorder, altered signaling can contribute to the symptomatology. The vagus nerve plays a role in stress response, and stress is a known exacerbating factor for IBS. Reduced vagal tone can influence intestinal sensitivity and motility.
- Visceral Hypersensitivity: Dysfunction in vagus nerve signaling

can contribute to heightened pain sensitivity in the gut. The vagus nerve modulates pain signaling in the gut; thus, its dysfunction can lead to an exaggerated pain response to normal intestinal processes.

- Functional Dyspepsia: Vagus nerve dysfunction may contribute to symptoms like bloating and discomfort. Altered vagal signaling can lead to poor coordination between the stomach and small intestine, resulting in symptoms that overlap with dyspepsia.

In conclusion, the vagus nerve plays multifaceted roles in the small intestine's functioning, ensuring efficient digestion and absorption, protecting the gut lining, and facilitating essential communication between the gut and the brain. The vagus nerve's health and function can directly influence the overall health and functioning of the digestive system.

References

1. Cryan, J.F., O'Riordan, K.J., Cowan, C.S.M., Sandhu, K.V., Bastiaanssen, T.F.S., Boehme, M., Codagnone, M.G., Cussotto, S., Fulling, C., Golubeva, A.V., Guzzetta, K.E., Jaggar, M., Long-Smith, C.M., Lyte, J.M., Martin, J.A., Molinero-Perez, A., Moloney, G., Morelli, E., Morillas, E., O'Connor, R., Cruz-Pereira, J.S., Peterson, V.L., Rea, K., Ritz, N.L., Sherwin, E., Spichak, S., Teichman, E.M., van de Wouw, M., Ventura-Silva, A.P., Wallace-Fitzsimons, S.E., Hyland, N., Clarke, G., and Dinan, T.G., 2019. 'The Microbiota-Gut-Brain Axis', Physiol Rev, 99(4), pp.1877.

2. Margolis, K.G., Cryan, J.F., and Mayer, E.A., 2021. 'The Microbiota-Gut-Brain Axis: From Motility to Mood', Gastroenterology, 160(5), pp.1486-1501. doi: 10.1053/j.gastro.2020.10.066.

3. Qu, T., Han, W., Niu, J., Tong, J., and de Araujo, I.E., 2019. 'On the roles of the Duodenum and the Vagus nerve in learned nutrient preferences', Appetite, 139, pp.145-151. doi: 10.1016/j.appet.2019.04.014.

4. Ross, R.C., He, Y., Townsend, R.L., Schauer, P.R., Berthoud, H.R., Morrison, C.D., and Albaugh, V.L., 2023. 'The Vagus Nerve Mediates Gut-Brain Response to Duodenal Nutrient Administration', Am Surg, 89(8), pp.3600-3602. doi: 10.1177/00031348231161680.

5. Van Der Zanden, E.P., Boeckxstaens, G.E., and de Jonge, W.J., 2009. 'The vagus nerve as a modulator of intestinal inflammation', Neurogastroenterol Motil, 21(1), pp.6-17. doi: 10.1111/j.1365-2982.2008.01252.x.

6. Zhang, X., Fogel, R., and Renehan, W.E., 1992. 'Physiology and morphology of neurons in the dorsal motor nucleus of the vagus and the nucleus of the solitary tract that are sensitive to distension of the small intestine', J Comp Neurol, 323(3), pp.432-448. doi: 10.1002/cne.903230310.

Chapter 12
The Vagus Nerve and the Liver

The vagus nerve, primarily known for its vast reach and influence over multiple organ systems, does not have as direct and pronounced an influence on the liver as it does on some other organs like the heart, stomach, or lungs. However, it does play roles in indirect mechanisms that affect liver function:

1. Glycogen Synthesis and Breakdown:
- Glucose Homeostasis: Through complex neuro-hormonal pathways, the vagus nerve plays a role in glucose metabolism, influencing both glycogen synthesis and its breakdown, known as glycogenolysis, in the liver.
- Glycogenolysis: Vagal stimulation can also influence the breakdown of glycogen into glucose, a process known as glycogenolysis.

2. Hepatic Blood Flow Regulation:
- The vagus nerve can affect the hepatic artery's blood flow, thereby potentially influencing the amount of oxygen and nutrients delivered to liver cells.

3. Influence on Bile Production:
- While the exact mechanisms remain uncertain, evidence suggests that the vagus nerve can impact bile production in the liver.. Bile is essential for the emulsification and digestion of fats in the small intestine.

4. Role in Hepatic Regeneration:
- There's some evidence that vagal stimulation might promote liver regeneration after hepatic injury. The exact mechanisms of this influence are still under investigation.

5. Gut-Liver Axis and Immune Regulation:
- The vagus nerve is integral to the gut-brain axis, indirectly influencing the liver due to its role in detoxifying substances and processing gut-absorbed nutrients.
- Vagal stimulation can potentially modulate immune responses in the liver, especially given its known anti-inflammatory effects in other organ systems.

6. Potential Role in Fatty Liver Disease:
- Some research suggests that the vagus nerve might play a role in the pathogenesis and progression of non-alcoholic fatty liver disease (NAFLD). Vagal influence on lipid metabolism and inflammatory pathways could be factors.

7. Hepatic Gluconeogenesis:
- The liver can produce glucose from non-carbohydrate sources, a process called gluconeogenesis. Through its influence on various neuro-hormonal pathways, the vagus nerve might have a modulatory effect on this process.

8. Hepatic Lipogenesis:
- Lipogenesis is the process of converting acetyl-CoA into fatty acids in the liver. The vagus nerve, through its complex interactions with hormonal pathways, might play a role in influencing this metabolic pathway.

Clinical Significance of Vagus Nerve Dysfunction:
- Hepatic Steatosis (Fatty Liver): The vagus nerve is involved in regulating lipid metabolism. Its dysfunction may contribute to altered lipid storage in hepatocytes. Poor vagal tone could impact the liver's ability to properly manage lipids, contributing to the accumulation of fat in liver cells.
- Impaired Gluconeogenesis: The vagus nerve modulates liver glucose production through its parasympathetic signaling pathways. Dysfunction may lead to inefficient regulation of gluconeogenesis,

THE VAGUS NERVE AND THE LIVER

which could result in issues related to blood sugar levels.

- Altered Detoxification Processes: The vagus nerve plays a role in signaling liver functions, including detoxification processes. Dysfunction might impair the liver's ability to detoxify certain substances, possibly leading to increased toxicity in the body.

- Liver Cirrhosis and Portal Hypertension: While not directly caused by vagus nerve dysfunction, impaired vagal activity may exacerbate the autonomic imbalance seen in cirrhosis. Reduced vagal signaling might impair hepatic blood flow regulation, potentially aggravating conditions like portal hypertension.

- Hepatic Encephalopathy: Vagus nerve dysfunction can contribute to altered neurotransmitter levels that may exacerbate hepatic encephalopathy symptoms. Disruption in vagus nerve signaling may impact liver-brain communications and exacerbate neurocognitive symptoms.

- Bile Secretion Impairment: The vagus nerve contributes to the regulation of bile secretion, which is crucial for fat digestion. Vagal dysfunction could lead to an imbalance in bile secretion, affecting fat metabolism and absorption.

- Inflammation and Liver Injury: The vagus nerve has anti-inflammatory effects that can modulate liver inflammation. Reduced vagal activity might result in poorly regulated inflammation, potentially exacerbating liver injury in conditions such as hepatitis.

- Drug Metabolism: The vagus nerve modulates certain enzyme activities in the liver. Dysfunction could lead to altered drug metabolism rates, affecting drug efficacy or increasing toxicity.

It's important to note that many of these conditions can arise from a multitude of factors. Vagus nerve dysfunction is just one potential contributor and should not be considered the sole cause without appropriate medical evaluation. Always consult healthcare providers for accurate diagnosis and treatment.

To sum up, while the vagus nerve's direct influence on the liver isn't as pronounced as its effect on some other organs, its indirect roles, particularly through the gut-liver axis and its influence on metabolic and immune pathways, mean that it's still crucial for liver health and function. Research in this area continues to uncover the nuances of the vagus nerve's role in hepatic physiology.

References

1. Ding, J.H., Jin, Z., Yang, X.X., Lou, J., Shan, W.X., Hu, Y.X., Du, Q., Liao, Q.S., Xie, R. and Xu, J.Y., 2020. 'Role of gut microbiota via the gut-liver-brain axis in digestive diseases', World J Gastroenterol, 26(40), pp.6141-6162. doi: 10.3748/wjg.v26.i40.6141.

2. Matsubara, Y., Kiyohara, H., Teratani, T., Mikami, Y. and Kanai, T., 2022. 'Organ and brain crosstalk: The liver-brain axis in gastrointestinal, liver, and pancreatic diseases', Neuropharmacology, 205, p.108915. doi: 10.1016/j.neuropharm.2021.108915.

3. Metz, C.N. and Pavlov, V.A., 2018. 'Vagus nerve cholinergic circuitry to the liver and the gastrointestinal tract in the neuroimmune communicatome', Am J Physiol Gastrointest Liver Physiol, 315(5), pp.G651-G658. doi: 10.1152/ajpgi.00195.2018

4. Milosevic, I., Vujovic, A., Barac, A., Djelic, M., Korac, M., Radovanovic Spurnic, A., Gmizic, I., Stevanovic, O., Djordjevic, V., Lekic, N., Russo, E. and Amedei, A., 2019. 'Gut-Liver Axis, Gut Microbiota, and Its Modulation in the Management of Liver Diseases: A Review of the Literature', Int J Mol Sci, 20(2), p.395. doi: 10.3390/ijms20020395.

Chapter 13
The Vagus Nerve and the Gallbladder

The vagus nerve, as part of the parasympathetic nervous system, has a role in many visceral functions. Its influence over the gallbladder, like with several other organs, is through a mix of direct and indirect pathways:

1. Gallbladder Contraction:

Bile Release: One of the primary functions of the gallbladder is to store and concentrate bile, which is produced by the liver. Upon the ingestion of a meal, especially one containing fats, the gallbladder contracts to release this bile into the duodenum. The vagus nerve has been suggested to play a role in this process, with vagal stimulation promoting gallbladder contraction.

2. CCK Release:

Cholecystokinin (CCK) Stimulation: When fatty or protein-rich chyme enters the duodenum, the enteroendocrine cells of the small intestine release CCK. CCK is a major stimulant for gallbladder contraction. The vagus nerve indirectly influences this process by modulating CCK release. Vagal stimulation enhances the sensitivity of the gallbladder to CCK.

3. Gut-Brain Axis Communication:

Sensory Feedback: The vagus nerve provides sensory feedback from the gallbladder to the central nervous system. Any distension or discomfort in the gallbladder can be relayed via the vagus, playing a role in the reflex pathways that regulate gallbladder function.

4. Protection against Gallstones:

Vagus nerve-modulated regular emptying and filling of the gallbladder can act as a protective measure against gallstone formation. Bile stagnation can result in the precipitation of cholesterol or bilirubin, culminating in stone formation.

5. Anti-inflammatory Effects:

The vagus nerve is known for its anti-inflammatory properties in various organs. While direct evidence of its role in gallbladder inflammation (cholecystitis) is limited, the potential exists for vagal stimulation to modulate inflammatory responses in the gallbladder.

Clinical Significance of Vagus Nerve Dysfunction:
- Gallbladder Dyskinesia (Biliary Dyskinesia): The vagus nerve plays a role in coordinating gallbladder contractions to release bile. Dysfunction of the vagus nerve may lead to irregular or ineffective gallbladder contractions, contributing to symptoms like pain and indigestion.
- Gallstones (Cholelithiasis): While gallstones have multiple contributing factors, altered vagus nerve function could potentially affect bile secretion and gallbladder emptying. If the gallbladder doesn't empty efficiently due to vagus nerve dysfunction, bile could become concentrated and lead to gallstone formation.
- Cholecystitis (Inflamed Gallbladder): The vagus nerve has anti-inflammatory effects that can influence inflammation within the gallbladder. Impaired vagal activity could potentially exacerbate the inflammatory process seen in conditions like cholecystitis.
- Postcholecystectomy Syndrome: Removal of the gallbladder can sometimes result in changes to vagus nerve signaling related to digestion. Post-surgical changes might disrupt vagal activity, leading to symptoms such as bloating, pain, and diarrhea after gallbladder removal.
- Altered Bile Composition: The vagus nerve influences bile secretion and composition through its regulatory effects. Dysfunction may alter bile composition, which could have downstream effects like poor fat digestion or increased risk of stone formation.

- Delayed Gastric Emptying: The vagus nerve also regulates stomach emptying, which has a downstream effect on gallbladder function. Delayed gastric emptying may disrupt the normal signaling pathways that trigger gallbladder contraction, affecting the overall digestive process.

- Gallbladder Polyps: While not directly linked, vagus nerve dysfunction might affect inflammatory processes that could potentially contribute to polyp formation. Altered vagal signaling could exacerbate local inflammation and thereby contribute to polyp development.

- Sphincter of Oddi Dysfunction: The vagus nerve may influence the sphincter that controls the flow of bile and pancreatic juices into the small intestine. Dysfunction can lead to irregularities in sphincter function, affecting bile flow and possibly contributing to pain and digestive issues.

Please note that these are potential scenarios where vagus nerve dysfunction could have an effect on gallbladder conditions. They are not definitive causes and should not replace professional medical advice. Always consult healthcare providers for accurate diagnosis and appropriate treatment.

In conclusion, the vagus nerve plays a role in gallbladder function, mainly through its influence on gallbladder contractions and the release of bile into the duodenum. Additionally, its indirect effects through the modulation of bile production in the liver and its potential anti-inflammatory properties further underline its importance in gallbladder health.

References

1. Ding, J.H., Jin, Z., Yang, X.X., Lou, J., Shan, W.X., Hu, Y.X., Du, Q., Liao, Q.S., Xie, R. and Xu, J.Y., 2020. 'Role of gut microbiota via the gut-liver-brain axis in digestive diseases', World J Gastroenterol, 26(40), pp.6141-6162. doi: 10.3748/wjg.v26.i40.6141. PMID: 33177790; PMCID: PMC7596643.

2. Magee, D.F., Naruse, S. and Pap, A., 1984. 'Vagal control of gallbladder contraction', J Physiol, 355, pp.65-70. doi: 10.1113/jphysiol.1984.sp015402.

3. Matsubara, Y., Kiyohara, H., Teratani, T., Mikami, Y. and Kanai, T., 2022. 'Organ and brain crosstalk: The liver-brain axis in gastrointestinal, liver, and pancreatic diseases', Neuropharmacology, 205, p.108915. doi: 10.1016/j.neuropharm.2021.108915. Epub 2021 Dec 15. PMID: 34919906.

4. Metz, C.N. and Pavlov, V.A., 2018. 'Vagus nerve cholinergic circuitry to the liver and the gastrointestinal tract in the neuroimmune communicatome', Am J Physiol Gastrointest Liver Physiol, 315(5), pp.G651-G658. doi: 10.1152/ajpgi.00195.2018. PMID: 30001146; PMCID: PMC6293249.

5. Milosevic, I., Vujovic, A., Barac, A., Djelic, M., Korac, M., Radovanovic Spurnic, A., Gmizic, I., Stevanovic, O., Djordjevic, V., Lekic, N., Russo, E. and Amedei, A., 2019. 'Gut-Liver Axis, Gut Microbiota, and Its Modulation in the Management of Liver Diseases: A Review of the Literature', Int J Mol Sci, 20(2), p.395. doi: 10.3390/ijms20020395. PMID: 30658519; PMCID: PMC6358912.

Chapter 14
The Vagus Nerve and the Large Intestine

The vagus nerve, known for its expansive reach throughout the body, does play roles in the functioning of the large intestine, though its influence is more pronounced in the upper parts of the gastrointestinal tract. Here's a breakdown of the vagus nerve's interactions with the large intestine:

1. Motility:

Haustral Contractions: Haustra are the sac-like pouches in the large intestine. These pouches undergo contractions to help mix and propel fecal material. The vagus nerve plays a role, though less dominant than in the small intestine, in modulating these contractions, ensuring that the contents move steadily towards the rectum.

2. Reflexes:

Gastrocolic Reflex: This is a physiologic reflex that occurs after eating, where the presence of food in the stomach triggers motility in the colon, preparing the large intestine for the arrival of chyme. The vagus nerve is involved in mediating this reflex.

Defecation Reflex: While primarily governed by local reflexes and the sacral parasympathetic system, the vagus nerve can play a role in initiating the urge to defecate when the rectum is distended.

3. Secretion:

Mucus Production: Goblet cells in the lining of the large intestine produce mucus, which helps lubricate fecal matter and protect the intestinal lining. The vagus nerve might play a role in modulating mucus secretion, though this role is not as well-defined as in other parts of the digestive tract.

4. Gut-Brain Communication:

Sensory Feedback: The vagus nerve relays sensory information from the large intestine back to the brain. This feedback can provide information about distension, inflammation, or other pathologies.

Gut-Brain Axis: The vagus nerve is a major component of the gut-brain axis, which establishes bidirectional communication between the gastrointestinal tract and the central nervous system. This has implications not just for motility and secretion, but also for mood and overall well-being.

5. Anti-inflammatory Properties:

Modulation of Immune Responses: The vagus nerve can influence immune responses in the gut. In the context of inflammatory bowel diseases, like ulcerative colitis which primarily affects the large intestine, there's interest in the potential anti-inflammatory effects of vagal stimulation.

6. Microbiome Interactions:

Feedback Mechanisms: The large intestine houses a significant portion of the gut microbiota. The vagus nerve can detect changes or imbalances in this microbiota and relay that information to the brain, which can then respond with necessary regulatory actions.

Clinical Significance of Vagus Nerve Dysfunction:

- Constipation: The vagus nerve plays a role in stimulating peristaltic movements in the large intestine. Reduced vagal activity may lead to slowed intestinal motility, contributing to constipation.

- Irritable Bowel Syndrome (IBS): Vagus nerve dysfunction may exacerbate symptoms such as irregular bowel movements, bloating, and abdominal pain. Poor vagal tone may affect stress response, intestinal sensitivity, and motility, all of which can contribute to IBS symptoms.

- Colonic Inertia: This is a condition characterized by a lack of rhythmic contractions in the colon. Vagus nerve dysfunction could lead to impaired signaling for peristalsis, contributing to colonic inertia.

- Megacolon: Vagal dysfunction can result in decreased colonic motility. The lack of appropriate vagal stimulation could lead to dilation and enlargement of the colon (megacolon).

- Diverticulitis: Although not a direct cause, vagus nerve dysfunction could potentially exacerbate symptoms by affecting gut motility. Poor motility can contribute to fecal stagnation, raising the risk of diverticular inflammation.

- Stress-induced Flare-ups in Inflammatory Bowel Disease (IBD): The vagus nerve is involved in stress response, which can affect the severity of IBD symptoms. Poor vagal tone can contribute to stress-induced exacerbations in conditions like Crohn's disease and ulcerative colitis.

- Gut Microbiota Imbalance: Vagus nerve activity can influence the gut-brain axis and, by extension, the gut microbiota. Dysfunction might contribute to an imbalance in gut bacteria, affecting colon health and function indirectly.

- Visceral Hypersensitivity: Visceral hypersensitivity refers to an increased pain sensitivity in the gut, often perceived when there's no clear cause for the pain. Vagus nerve dysfunction can contribute to heightened pain sensitivity in the gut. Reduced vagal activity may lead to an exaggerated pain response to normal or minimally invasive colonic stimuli.

- Postoperative Ileus: Surgical procedures can sometimes impact vagus nerve function. This disruption can lead to inhibited colonic motility, resulting in postoperative ileus, a condition where the intestine temporarily stops functioning.

As always, these conditions can have multiple etiologies, and vagus nerve dysfunction should not be considered the sole cause. Consult healthcare providers for accurate diagnosis and treatment.

In summary, while the vagus nerve's influence on the large intestine isn't as extensive as on some other organs, it still has a notable role in motility, secretion, and the complex gut-brain communication system. This intricate relationship underscores the importance of the vagus nerve in maintaining gut health and overall physiological balance.

References

1. Ahn, E.H., Kang, S.S., Liu, X., Chen, G., Zhang, Z., Chandrasekharan, B., Alam, A.M., Neish, A.S., Cao, X. and Ye, K., 2020. 'Initiation of Parkinson's disease from gut to brain by δ-secretase', Cell Res, 30(1), pp.70-87. doi: 10.1038/s41422-019-0241-9. PMID: 31649329; PMCID: PMC6951265.

2. Baquiran, M. and Bordoni, B., 2023. 'Anatomy, Head and Neck: Anterior Vagus Nerve', StatPearls, Treasure Island (FL): StatPearls Publishing. PMID: 31613476.

3. Furness, J.B., Callaghan, B.P., Rivera, L.R. and Cho, H.J., 2014. 'The enteric nervous system and gastrointestinal innervation: integrated local and central control', Adv Exp Med Biol, 817, pp.39-71. doi: 10.1007/978-1-4939-0897-4_3. PMID: 24997029.

4. Mayer, E.A., Nance, K. and Chen, S., 2022. 'The Gut-Brain Axis', Annu Rev Med, 73, pp.439-453. doi: 10.1146/annurev-med-042320-014032. Epub 2021 Oct 20. PMID: 34669431.

5. Meroni, E., Stakenborg, N., Gomez-Pinilla, P.J., Stakenborg, M., Aguilera-Lizarraga, J., Florens, M., Delfini, M., de Simone, V., De Hertogh, G., Goverse, G., Matteoli, G. and Boeckxstaens, G.E., 2021. 'Vagus Nerve Stimulation Promotes Epithelial Proliferation and Controls Colon Monocyte Infiltration During DSS-Induced Colitis', Front Med (Lausanne), 8, p.694268. doi: 10.3389/fmed.2021.694268. PMID: 34307422; PMCID: PMC8292675.

6. Socała, K., Doboszewska, U., Szopa, A., Serefko, A., Włodarczyk, M., Zielińska, A., Poleszak, E., Fichna, J. and Wlaź, P., 2021. 'The role of microbiota-gut-brain axis in neuropsychiatric and neurological disorders', Pharmacol Res, 172, p.105840. doi: 10.1016/j.phrs.2021.105840. Epub 2021 Aug 24. PMID: 34450312.

Chapter 15
The Vagus Nerve and the Kidneys

The kidneys, crucial organs for fluid and electrolyte balance as well as waste filtration, aren't as directly influenced by the vagus nerve as many of the other organs we've discussed. However, the vagus nerve, due to its extensive connectivity and its regulatory roles, does have some interactions with the kidneys, both directly and indirectly:

1. Renal Blood Flow Regulation:

The vagus nerve plays a role in the overall regulation of blood pressure and heart rate. While it doesn't directly innervate the kidneys to the same degree as it does some other organs, any alteration in blood pressure can indirectly affect renal blood flow.

2. Natriuresis:

Natriuresis is the process of sodium excretion in the urine. There is evidence from some studies to suggest that vagal stimulation can influence natriuresis, though the mechanism is not entirely clear.

3. Inflammatory Modulation:

Anti-inflammatory Effects: As with other organs, the vagus nerve has anti-inflammatory effects, which have potential implications for renal health. In conditions like acute kidney injury or chronic kidney disease, where inflammation plays a role, vagal stimulation might provide protective or therapeutic benefits.

4. Neuro-Hormonal Pathways:

The kidneys play a central role in the renin-angiotensin-aldosterone system (RAAS), which regulates blood pressure, fluid balance, and sodium balance.

While the vagus nerve doesn't directly control RAAS, its influence over the heart and blood vessels can have secondary effects on this system.

5. Sensory Feedback:

As with other organs, the vagus nerve might help relay sensory information from the kidneys back to the brain, particularly under conditions of stress or injury.

6. Gut-Kidney Axis:

While the gut-brain axis mediated by the vagus is more commonly discussed, there's also a gut-kidney axis. Changes in gut health can influence kidney health, and vice versa. The vagus nerve, due to its influence over gut function, can indirectly play a role in this axis.

Clinical Significance of of Vagus Nerve Dysfunction:
- Chronic Kidney Disease (CKD): Vagus nerve dysfunction can contribute to systemic inflammation, a contributing factor in CKD. Reduced anti-inflammatory signaling via the vagus nerve may exacerbate the inflammatory processes that worsen CKD.
- Acute Kidney Injury (AKI): The vagus nerve has anti-inflammatory effects, which could potentially modulate the acute inflammatory response in AKI. Impaired vagal activity may reduce the kidney's resilience against acute stressors, like sepsis or ischemia, potentially aggravating AKI.
- Hypertension: While the sympathetic system is more directly involved, the vagus nerve plays a role in overall autonomic balance. Dysregulated vagal function could indirectly contribute to an imbalance in autonomic output, influencing blood pressure and, consequently, renal function.
- Proteinuria: Vagal dysfunction can contribute to systemic inflammation and endothelial dysfunction. Both these factors can affect the glomerular filtration barrier, potentially leading to proteinuria.
- Nephrolithiasis (Kidney Stones): Vagal activity is involved in overall

stress response, which may affect the excretion of stone-forming substances. Impaired vagal function could indirectly contribute to metabolic imbalances that facilitate stone formation.

- Diabetic Nephropathy: Vagal dysfunction may exacerbate systemic inflammation and oxidative stress, both of which are factors in diabetic nephropathy. Impaired anti-inflammatory signaling via the vagus nerve may exacerbate the pathophysiology of diabetic nephropathy.

- Renal Ischemia-Reperfusion Injury: The vagus nerve's anti-inflammatory role may modulate the extent of injury following ischemia and reperfusion. Reduced vagal activity might exacerbate the inflammatory response to reperfusion injury, potentially leading to more severe outcomes.

- Glomerulonephritis: The vagus nerve has anti-inflammatory properties that could influence the progression of glomerular diseases. Reduced vagal tone may contribute to a pro-inflammatory state, potentially worsening glomerulonephritis.

- Fluid and Electrolyte Balance: The vagus nerve contributes to overall homeostasis, including hormonal regulation. Although not directly influencing the kidneys, vagal dysfunction can alter systemic balance, affecting hormones like aldosterone and thereby impacting renal function.

As always, these are potential relationships between vagus nerve function and kidney conditions, and the presence of such a condition doesn't necessarily imply vagal dysfunction. It's essential to consult healthcare providers for a comprehensive diagnosis and appropriate treatment.

In conclusion, while the vagus nerve doesn't have as pronounced a direct influence over the kidneys as it does over, say, the heart or the digestive system, its indirect roles in regulating blood flow, modulating inflammation, and influencing neuro-hormonal pathways mean it still has implications for renal health.

References

1. Ariton, D.M., Jiménez-Balado, J., Maisterra, O., Pujadas, F., Soler, M.J. and Delgado, P., 2021. 'Diabetes, Albuminuria and the Kidney-Brain Axis', J Clin Med, 10(11), p.2364. doi: 10.3390/jcm10112364. PMID: 34072230; PMCID: PMC8198842.

2. Jarczyk, J., Yard, B.A. and Hoeger, S., 2019. 'The Cholinergic Anti-Inflammatory Pathway as a Conceptual Framework to Treat Inflammation-Mediated Renal Injury', Kidney Blood Press Res, 44(4), pp.435-448. doi: 10.1159/000500920. Epub 2019 Jul 15. PMID: 31307039.

3. Tanaka, S. and Okusa, M.D., 2020. 'Crosstalk between the nervous system and the kidney', Kidney Int, 97(3), pp.466-476. doi: 10.1016/j.kint.2019.10.032. Epub 2019 Nov 22. PMID: 32001065; PMCID: PMC7039752.

4. Yang, T., Richards, E.M., Pepine, C.J. and Raizada, M.K., 2018. 'The gut microbiota and the brain-gut-kidney axis in hypertension and chronic kidney disease', Nat Rev Nephrol, 14(7), pp.442-456. doi: 10.1038/s41581-018-0018-2. PMID: 29760448; PMCID: PMC6385605.

Chapter 16
The Vagus Nerve and the Bladder and Urethra

The urinary bladder and the urethra are primarily influenced by the autonomic nervous system, specifically the sympathetic and parasympathetic divisions. The vagus nerve, being a major component of the parasympathetic nervous system, has some influence on these structures, but it's essential to note that the primary parasympathetic innervation to the bladder and urethra comes from the sacral part of the spinal cord (S2-S4) via the pelvic splanchnic nerves. However, the vagus nerve can still have indirect and modulatory effects:

1. Bladder Filling and Emptying:

While the pelvic splanchnic nerves are primarily responsible for bladder contraction during micturition, the vagus nerve might play a role in modulating the sensation of bladder fullness or the urge to urinate.

2. Urethral Sphincter Control:

The urethral sphincter's opening and closing are crucial for retaining and releasing urine. Sympathetic fibers generally keep the sphincter closed, and parasympathetic fibers aid in its relaxation for micturition. The vagus nerve can influence this dynamic balance, particularly in sensing and signaling the need to void.

3. Reflex Arcs:

The micturition reflex, which involves both the bladder and urethra, is a coordinated response that's influenced by higher centers in the brain and brainstem. The vagus nerve, due to its extensive brainstem connections, might be involved in modulating this reflex, especially under conditions of stress or other stimuli.

4. Sensory Feedback:

The vagus nerve could help in relaying sensory information from the bladder and urethra back to the brain. This might be particularly relevant in situations like bladder infections, where there's increased sensitivity and urgency.

5. Anti-inflammatory Role:

Given its known anti-inflammatory effects in various organs, the vagus nerve might offer protective benefits in the context of urinary tract infections or interstitial cystitis (a chronic bladder condition).

6. Gut-Bladder Communication:

The vagus nerve plays a significant role in gut function. There's a potential for gut-bladder crosstalk, especially since both systems share some common neural pathways. Disturbances in one can influence the other.

7. Influence on Blood Flow:

By modulating blood pressure and influencing vasodilation or vasoconstriction, the vagus nerve can indirectly impact the blood flow to the bladder and urethra, which can have implications during inflammation or injury.

Clinical Significance of of Vagus Nerve Dysfunction:
- Overactive Bladder (OAB): Vagal dysfunction could disrupt the overall autonomic regulation, potentially influencing bladder control. Altered autonomic balance may exacerbate the symptoms of urgency and frequency seen in OAB.
- Interstitial Cystitis/Bladder Pain Syndrome: The vagus nerve has anti-inflammatory properties that may be protective in conditions like interstitial cystitis. Reduced vagal tone could exacerbate the inflammatory environment, worsening the symptoms of pain and urgency.
- Urinary Retention: Though not directly innervating the bladder, the vagus nerve can affect overall autonomic balance, which might

impact bladder emptying. Altered autonomic regulation could contribute to an imbalance in detrusor muscle function, leading to urinary retention.

- Neurogenic Bladder: The vagus nerve plays a role in overall nervous system function, and dysfunction may indirectly affect conditions like neurogenic bladder. Altered neural control due to vagal dysfunction could exacerbate symptoms of either urinary retention or incontinence in neurogenic bladder cases.

- Stress-Induced Incontinence: The vagus nerve has a role in stress response and may impact stress-induced urinary symptoms. Vagal imbalance may contribute to heightened stress reactions, which can exacerbate stress-induced incontinence.

- Detrusor Overactivity: Altered autonomic balance due to vagal dysfunction could contribute to overactivity of the detrusor muscle. Imbalanced autonomic regulation could lead to involuntary detrusor contractions, causing urgency and frequency.

- Detrusor Underactivity: Vagal dysfunction might indirectly affect detrusor muscle contractility. Reduced overall autonomic regulation could contribute to weak or absent detrusor contractions, resulting in incomplete bladder emptying.

- Urethral Syndrome: Though not directly involved, vagus nerve dysfunction might exacerbate symptoms like urethral discomfort or frequency. Altered autonomic balance could affect sensitivity or muscle tone in the urethra.

- Urethral Stricture: Vagus nerve function can affect overall tissue healing and inflammation. Impaired vagal activity could potentially slow down the healing process or exacerbate inflammation, complicating urethral strictures.

As always, these are only potential relationships between vagus nerve dysfunction and bladder and urethral conditions. For an accurate diagnosis and appropriate treatment, it's crucial to consult healthcare providers.

To sum it up, the vagus nerve's influence over the bladder and urethra is more modulatory and indirect when compared to its direct roles in other organs. Still, its involvement in reflex arcs, sensory feedback, and potential anti-inflammatory roles underscores its importance in the overall urinary function.

References

1. Barbe, M.F., Gomez-Amaya, S., Braverman, A.S., Brown, J.M., Lamarre, N.S., Massicotte, V.S., Lewis, J.K., Dachert, S.R. and Ruggieri, M.R., Sr., 2017. 'Evidence of vagus nerve sprouting to innervate the urinary bladder and clitoris in a canine model of lower motoneuron lesioned bladder', Neurourol Urodyn, 36(1), pp.91-97. doi: 10.1002/nau.22904. Epub 2015 Oct 9. PMID: 26452068; PMCID: PMC4826634.

2. Hassan, A.A., Hicks, M.N., Walters, G.E. and Mary, D.A., 1987. 'Effect on efferent cardiac vagal nerve fibres of distension of the urinary bladder in the dog', Q J Exp Physiol, 72(4), pp.473-481. doi: 10.1113/expphysiol.1987.sp003089. PMID: 3423196.

3. Jung, J., Kim, A. and Yang, S.H., 2023. 'The Innovative Approach in Functional Bladder Disorders: The Communication Between Bladder and Brain-Gut Axis', Int Neurourol J, 27(1), pp.15-22. doi: 10.5213/inj.2346036.018. Epub 2023 Mar 31. PMID: 37015721; PMCID: PMC10072998.

4. Leue, C., Kruimel, J., Vrijens, D., Masclee, A., van Os, J. and van Koeveringe, G., 2017. 'Functional urological disorders: a sensitized defence response in the bladder-gut-brain axis', Nat Rev Urol, 14(3), pp.153-163. doi: 10.1038/nrurol.2016.227. Epub 2016 Dec 6. PMID: 27922040.

Chapter 17
The Vagus Nerve and the Spleen

The vagus nerve's relationship with the spleen is a compelling topic, especially in the context of the inflammatory reflex and the body's immune response. Here's an in-depth look at the connection between the vagus nerve and the spleen:

Inflammatory Reflex:

The vagus nerve plays a key role in the inflammatory reflex, a physiological mechanism through which the central nervous system regulates the immune response. When there's an inflammatory event in the body, cytokines and other inflammatory mediators are produced. These signals can be detected by the afferent (sensory) fibers of the vagus nerve.

Upon receiving these signals, the central nervous system activates the efferent (motor) fibers of the vagus nerve, which then send signals to various organs involved in the immune response, including the spleen.

Spleen's Role in Immunity:

The spleen is a vital organ in the immune system. It produces immune cells (like B and T cells), filters old and damaged red blood cells, and stores platelets. The spleen also produces antibodies and removes bacteria and other pathogens from the blood.

When the inflammatory reflex is triggered, the vagus nerve communicates with the spleen to modulate its immune activity. This involves a complex interplay between neurons, immune cells, and cytokines.

THE VAGUS NERVE

Cholinergic Anti-inflammatory Pathway:

This pathway is a significant mechanism by which the vagus nerve suppresses inflammation. Activation of the vagus nerve leads to the release of acetylcholine, a neurotransmitter. Acetylcholine interacts with immune cells, specifically macrophages, and inhibits the release of pro-inflammatory cytokines like TNF-alpha. More in the following chapters.

Clinical Implications of Vagus Nerve Dysfunction:
- Splenomegaly (Enlarged Spleen): The vagus nerve's anti-inflammatory actions may affect the condition of an enlarged spleen. Reduced vagal tone could exacerbate underlying inflammatory conditions that lead to splenomegaly.

- Splenic Infarction (Disrupted Splenic Blood Flow): Vagal dysfunction might impact the body's overall inflammatory response to tissue damage. Reduced anti-inflammatory signaling may complicate the healing or recovery process after splenic infarction.

- Autoimmune Conditions Affecting the Spleen: Vagal nerve activity has been linked to the modulation of immune responses. Poor vagal tone may contribute to immune dysregulation, affecting conditions like autoimmune hemolytic anemia where the spleen is involved.

- Hypersplenism: Vagus nerve dysfunction could potentially affect the rate of blood cell destruction in the spleen. Imbalanced autonomic output could exacerbate conditions of hypersplenism, where the spleen removes blood cells at an abnormally high rate.

- Sepsis-Induced Splenic Dysfunction: The vagus nerve has a role in modulating the systemic inflammatory response, which is heightened in sepsis. Poor vagal activity might worsen the splenic dysfunction commonly seen in septic conditions.

- Splenic Rupture: While the vagus nerve is not directly involved in traumatic injuries, its role in inflammation and healing could impact recovery. Reduced vagal activity could potentially slow down the healing process and complicate recovery from a splenic rupture.

- Postsplenectomy Infection Risk: The vagus nerve plays a role in immune regulation, and its dysfunction could potentially affect susceptibility to infections. Reduced vagal tone could weaken the immune response, making post-splenectomy patients more vulnerable to infections.

- Splenic Cysts and Tumors: Vagal tone may have an indirect impact on inflammatory environments conducive to cyst or tumor formation. Poor vagal activity could contribute to systemic inflammation, affecting the condition or progression of splenic cysts or tumors.

- Hematological Conditions: Vagal nerve dysfunction might impact the spleen's role in filtering blood and recycling red blood cells. Altered autonomic function may contribute to or exacerbate hematological conditions where the spleen plays a role, such as certain types of anemia.

As always, these conditions can have multiple etiologies, and vagus nerve dysfunction should not be considered the sole cause. Consult healthcare providers for accurate diagnosis and treatment.

In summary, the vagus nerve doesn't directly innervate the spleen, but it profoundly influences its function through the inflammatory reflex and the cholinergic anti-inflammatory pathway. This interaction holds promise for new therapeutic strategies targeting a range of inflammatory conditions.

References

1. Bonaz, B., Sinniger, V., and Pellissier, S., 2017. 'The Vagus Nerve in the Neuro-Immune Axis: Implications in the Pathology of the Gastrointestinal Tract', Front Immunol, 8, p.1452. doi: 10.3389/fimmu.2017.01452. PMID: 29163522; PMCID: PMC5673632.

2. Simon, T., Kirk, J., Dolezalova, N., Guyot, M., Panzolini, C., Bondue, A., Lavergne, J., Hugues, S., Hypolite, N., Saeb-Parsy, K., Perkins, J., Macia, E., Sridhar, A., Vervoordeldonk, M.J., Glaichenhaus, N., Donegá, M., and Blancou, P., 2023. 'The cholinergic anti-inflammatory pathway inhibits inflammation without lymphocyte relay', Front Neurosci, 17, p.1125492. doi: 10.3389/fnins.2023.1125492. PMID: 37123375; PMCID: PMC10140439.

3. Wei, Y., Wang, T., Liao, L., Fan, X., Chang, L., and Hashimoto, K., 2022. 'Brain-spleen axis in health and diseases: A review and future perspective', Brain Res Bull, 182, pp.130-140. doi: 10.1016/j.brainresbull.2022.02.008. Epub 2022 Feb 12. PMID: 35157987.

Chapter 18
The Vagus Nerve and the Pancreas

The vagus nerve plays a role in the regulation of various physiological processes in the body, and the pancreas is no exception. The pancreas, an organ with both endocrine (hormonal) and exocrine (digestive) functions, is influenced by the vagus nerve primarily in its exocrine role, but there are also some implications for endocrine functions. Here's a detailed look:

Exocrine Function (Digestive Role):

The pancreas secretes digestive enzymes into the duodenum, the first part of the small intestine. These enzymes, which include amylase, lipase, and proteases, help in the digestion of carbohydrates, fats, and proteins, respectively.

    The vagus nerve plays a significant role in stimulating the pancreas to secrete these enzymes. When food is consumed, it stimulates receptors in the stomach and duodenum. These receptors relay signals to the brain, which in response activates the vagus nerve. The vagus nerve then stimulates the pancreas to release digestive enzymes to aid in the breakdown of the ingested food.

    Furthermore, the vagus nerve helps regulate the secretion of bicarbonate from the pancreas, which neutralizes the acidic chyme coming from the stomach, allowing for optimal enzymatic activity in the duodenum.

Endocrine Function (Hormonal Role):

The pancreas also has endocrine cells, known as the islets of Langerhans, which produce hormones such as insulin, glucagon, and somatostatin. These hormones play essential roles in regulating blood glucose levels.

While the primary regulation of these hormones is in response to blood glucose levels, the vagus nerve may have modulatory effects:

- Insulin: Some studies suggest that parasympathetic (vagal) activity can enhance insulin secretion in response to elevated blood glucose. This suggests that the vagus nerve might play a role in fine-tuning or amplifying the insulin response after meals.

- Glucagon: The relationship between the vagus nerve and glucagon secretion (a hormone that raises blood glucose) is more complex, with some evidence suggesting inhibitory effects.

Appetite Regulation:

The pancreas secretes another hormone called pancreatic polypeptide (PP). PP is believed to play a role in appetite regulation, with levels rising after a meal. The vagus nerve is involved in the secretion of PP, with vagal stimulation leading to increased PP secretion.

Clinical Implications of Vagus Nerve Dysfunction:

- Pancreatitis: The vagus nerve helps modulate inflammatory responses. Its dysfunction may contribute to the inflammation seen in pancreatitis. Reduced vagal activity may exacerbate the inflammatory pathways activated in pancreatitis, potentially worsening the condition.

- Diabetes Mellitus: The vagus nerve plays a role in glucose metabolism and insulin sensitivity. Altered vagal signaling could contribute to insulin resistance or inadequate insulin production, thereby impacting diabetes management.

- Exocrine Pancreatic Insufficiency: Vagal stimulation is involved in promoting the secretion of pancreatic enzymes. Dysfunction in vagal activity could contribute to insufficient enzyme production, exacerbating malabsorption issues.

- Hypoglycemia: The vagus nerve plays a role in regulating glucose levels and its dysfunction could affect hypoglycemic episodes. Poor vagal tone might lead to insufficient glucagon secretion, which is necessary to counterbalance low blood sugar.

- Gastrointestinal Motility Disorders: The vagus nerve regulates gastrointestinal motility, affecting the release of pancreatic juices into the small intestine. Vagal dysfunction could result in motility issues that indirectly impact pancreatic function, leading to symptoms like indigestion or malabsorption.

- Pancreatic Pseudocyst: The vagus nerve's anti-inflammatory properties may influence the formation and resolution of pancreatic pseudocysts. Reduced vagal activity may impair the body's ability to manage and resolve inflammation, possibly complicating pseudocyst conditions.

- Pancreatic Endocrine Tumors: Though not directly implicated, the vagus nerve's role in systemic inflammation may have an indirect effect on tumor growth. Altered vagal activity could potentially create a conducive environment for endocrine tumors within the pancreas.

- Pancreatic Abscess: The vagus nerve's immunomodulatory role might affect the body's response to infection. Reduced vagal signaling could impair immune function, complicating the management of pancreatic abscesses.

- Pancreatic Fistulas: The vagus nerve may have a role in tissue repair and healing, which could impact the healing of pancreatic fistulas. Poor vagal activity could potentially slow down the healing process, affecting the management of pancreatic fistulas.

As always, the involvement of the vagus nerve in these conditions is often complex and may not be the sole contributing factor. For accurate diagnosis and targeted treatment, consultation with healthcare providers is essential.

In summary, the vagus nerve plays a multifaceted role in the pancreatic function, influencing both digestive enzyme release and potentially modulating hormone secretion. Its intricate involvement in these processes highlights the importance of the brain-gut axis in maintaining physiological homeostasis.

References

1. Bruschetta, G. and Diano, S., 2019. 'Brain-to-pancreas signalling axis links nicotine and diabetes', Nature, 574(7778), pp.336-337. doi: 10.1038/d41586-019-02975-w. PMID: 31619783; PMCID: PMC7224251.

2. Curry, D.L., 1984. 'Reflex inhibition of insulin secretion: vagus nerve involvement via CNS', Am J Physiol, 247(6 Pt 1), pp.E827-32. doi: 10.1152/ajpendo.1984.247.6.E827. PMID: 6391200.

3. Desai, G.S., Zheng, C., Geetha, T., Mathews, S.T., White, B.D., Huggins, K.W., Zizza, C.A., Broderick, T.L., and Babu, J.R., 2014. 'The pancreas-brain axis: insight into disrupted mechanisms associating type 2 diabetes and Alzheimer's disease', J Alzheimers Dis, 42(2), pp.347-56. doi: 10.3233/JAD-140018. PMID: 24858405.

4. Helman, A., Marre, M., Bobbioni, E., Poussier, P., Reach, G., and Assan, R., 1982. 'The brain-islet axis: the nervous control of the endocrine pancreas', Diabete Metab, 8(1), pp.53-64. PMID: 6124468.

5. Makhmutova, M., Weitz, J., Tamayo, A., Pereira, E., Boulina, M., Almaça, J., Rodriguez-Diaz, R., and Caicedo, A., 2021. 'Pancreatic β-Cells Communicate With Vagal Sensory Neurons', Gastroenterology, 160(3), pp.875-888.e11. doi: 10.1053/j.gastro.2020.10.034. Epub 2020 Oct 26. PMID: 33121946; PMCID: PMC10009739.

Chapter 19
The Vagus Nerve and the Male Reproductive System

The vagus nerve, while extensive in its reach throughout the body, doesn't directly innervate the male reproductive organs in the pronounced way it does with some other organs. However, due to its overarching roles in autonomic regulation and signaling, it can have indirect or modulatory effects on male reproductive function.

1. Erectile Function: Erection is a parasympathetic response, primarily mediated by the pelvic nerves from sacral spinal segments (S2-S4). While the vagus nerve isn't the main nerve involved, its overall influence on parasympathetic tone could modulate erectile function.

2. Ejaculation: Ejaculation is mostly a sympathetic event. As with erection, although the vagus nerve isn't directly responsible for this function, its influence on autonomic balance may indirectly affect the process.

3. Sensory Feedback: Some studies indicate that the vagus nerve could be involved in transmitting sensory information from reproductive organs, notably the testes, back to the central nervous system. This may be particularly relevant in instances of trauma, inflammation, or other pathological conditions.

4. Testicular Blood Flow: If the vagus nerve can influence blood pressure and vascular tone, it might indirectly affect testicular blood flow, which is vital for spermatogenesis and overall testicular health.

5. Hormonal Regulation: The hypothalamus and pituitary gland, potentially influenced by the vagus nerve, are central in regulating male reproductive hormones, especially testosterone. The hypothalamus releases gonadotropin-

releasing hormone (GnRH), prompting the pituitary gland to release luteinizing hormone (LH) and follicle-stimulating hormone (FSH). LH and FSH then influence testicular function and spermatogenesis. Any vagal influence on the hypothalamus or pituitary could indirectly affect this hormonal axis.

6. Stress and Reproductive Health: Chronic stress can influence male reproductive health, affecting erectile function and spermatogenesis. As the vagus nerve has a role in the body's stress response, its modulation may have implications for reproductive health.

7. Anti-inflammatory Role: Like other organs, testes can face inflammatory conditions, such as orchitis. Given the known anti-inflammatory effects of the vagus nerve in various organs, it might offer some protective benefits against testicular inflammation.

Clinical Implications of Vagus Nerve Dysfunction:
- Erectile Dysfunction: The vagus nerve's role in stress modulation can indirectly affect erectile function, which is primarily mediated by parasympathetic activity. Excessive stress or anxiety, potentially exacerbated by vagal dysfunction, could interfere with the neural pathways required for an erection.

- Premature Ejaculation: While sympathetic nerves are primarily responsible for ejaculation, the vagus nerve's role in emotional regulation and stress response could have an indirect influence. Poor stress management due to vagal dysfunction might contribute to premature ejaculation.

- Testicular Pain: Vagal nerve dysfunction could potentially exacerbate chronic pain conditions, including testicular pain, by influencing inflammatory responses. Reduced anti-inflammatory signaling may contribute to chronic testicular pain syndromes.

- Reduced Libido: The vagus nerve has a role in modulating stress and anxiety, which can impact sexual desire. Excessive stress, potentially due to vagal dysfunction, can decrease libido by affecting testosterone levels and mental well-being.

THE VAGUS NERVE AND THE MALE REPRODUCTIVE SYSTEM

- Infertility: While the vagus nerve is not directly linked to sperm production, its role in systemic inflammation and stress modulation could indirectly affect fertility. Chronic stress or inflammation, potentially worsened by vagal dysfunction, can negatively impact sperm quality and count.

- Prostatitis: Chronic inflammation is a characteristic of some types of prostatitis, and the vagus nerve's anti-inflammatory role could potentially influence this. Vagal dysfunction could potentially worsen the symptoms of chronic prostatitis by affecting the body's inflammatory responses.

- Orchitis (Testicular Inflammation): The vagus nerve's anti-inflammatory properties might impact the severity or progression of orchitis. Inadequate vagal tone could contribute to a heightened inflammatory state, exacerbating orchitis.

- Varicocele: While the vagus nerve is not directly involved, its role in systemic inflammation might indirectly affect the condition. Poor vagal activity could contribute to an environment that aggravates varicocele symptoms.

- Hormonal Imbalance: Stress modulation via the vagus nerve can impact cortisol levels, which in turn can influence testosterone levels. Vagal dysfunction leading to chronic stress could result in hormonal imbalances affecting the male reproductive system.

As always, these conditions can have multiple etiologies, and vagus nerve dysfunction should not be considered the sole cause. For accurate diagnosis and treatment, consultation with healthcare providers is recommended.

In summary, while the vagus nerve doesn't have as pronounced a direct influence on the male reproductive organs as it does on some other organs, its indirect roles in hormonal regulation, blood flow, and autonomic balance can still have implications for male reproductive health.

References

1. Purves, D., Augustine, G., Fitzpatrick, D., Hall, W., LaMantia, A., Mooney, R., Platt, M. and White, L. (eds.), 2017. Neuroscience: 6th Edition. Oxford University Press USA.

2. Squire, L., Berg, D., Bloom, F.E., du Lac, S., Ghosh, A. and Spitzer, N.C. (eds.), 2012. Fundamental Neuroscience. 4th ed. Elsevier.

3. Llewellyn-Smith, I. J. and Verberne, A. J. M. (eds.) 2011. Central Regulation of Autonomic Functions, 2nd edn. Oxford University Press.

Chapter 20
The Vagus Nerve and the Female Reproductive System

The vagus nerve, as part of the parasympathetic division of the autonomic nervous system, plays roles in various body functions, including some aspects of reproductive health. However, direct innervation of the female reproductive organs by the vagus nerve is limited. Much of the innervation of the female reproductive organs is provided by the pelvic and hypogastric nerves. Still, the vagus nerve can have indirect or modulatory effects on female reproductive function:

1. Menstrual Cycle Regulation: The menstrual cycle is regulated by hormones released by the hypothalamus, pituitary gland, and the ovaries. While the vagus nerve doesn't directly control these hormones, its influence on the overall homeostasis of the body and the stress response might indirectly affect hormonal balance and menstrual regularity.

2. Uterine Blood Flow: As the vagus nerve can influence blood pressure and vascular tone, it might indirectly affect uterine blood flow, which is especially crucial during menstruation and pregnancy.

3. Pain Sensation: The vagus nerve might play a modulatory role in the perception of pain, including dysmenorrhea (painful menstruation). Vagal nerve stimulation has been researched for various pain management scenarios.

4. Stress and Reproductive Health: Chronic stress can impact the female reproductive system, influencing menstrual regularity, fertility, and overall reproductive health. The vagus nerve plays a role in the body's stress response, and its modulation might have implications for reproductive health.

5. Sexual Response: Sexual arousal and response involve a complex interplay between the sympathetic and parasympathetic nervous systems. While the vagus nerve isn't the primary nerve responsible for female sexual response, its role in parasympathetic signaling might have modulatory effects.

6. Pregnancy: The vagus nerve's roles in regulating heart rate, blood pressure, and gastrointestinal function can indirectly impact maternal health during pregnancy.

7. Anti-inflammatory Role: Given the known anti-inflammatory effects of the vagus nerve in various organs, it's possible that it offers some protective benefits in the context of inflammatory conditions of the female reproductive system, such as pelvic inflammatory disease.

8. Sensory Feedback: There's some evidence to suggest the vagus nerve might be involved in transmitting sensory information from the cervix and uterus back to the central nervous system. This might be particularly relevant during childbirth or conditions like endometriosis.

Clinical Implications of Vagus Nerve Dysfunction:
- Dysmenorrhea (Painful Menstruation): The vagus nerve's anti-inflammatory role may influence the severity of dysmenorrhea. Vagal dysfunction could contribute to a heightened inflammatory state, thereby exacerbating menstrual pain.
- Amenorrhea (Absent Menstruation): The vagus nerve's role in stress modulation could potentially influence amenorrhea. High stress levels, which could be worsened by vagal dysfunction, may interfere with hormonal regulation leading to missed periods.
- Premenstrual Syndrome (PMS): The vagus nerve helps in regulating mood and stress, factors that can contribute to PMS. Poor vagal function could exacerbate stress and mood swings, potentially worsening PMS symptoms.
- Endometriosis: The vagus nerve's anti-inflammatory role may have an indirect impact on endometriosis. Reduced anti-inflammatory signaling via the vagus nerve could potentially worsen endometriosis

symptoms.

- Polycystic Ovary Syndrome (PCOS): The vagus nerve has a role in systemic inflammation and metabolic homeostasis. Vagal dysfunction could contribute to the inflammatory and metabolic irregularities commonly found in PCOS.

- Infertility: Vagal activity affects overall stress and inflammation levels, which can indirectly impact fertility. Vagal dysfunction could exacerbate stress and inflammatory conditions, potentially affecting fertility.

- Ovarian Cysts: Vagal nerve's role in inflammation might affect the condition indirectly. Poor vagal activity could contribute to an inflammatory environment that may affect ovarian cyst formation or exacerbation.

- Sexual Dysfunction: The vagus nerve is involved in stress regulation, which can indirectly impact sexual function. Dysfunction in the vagus nerve could contribute to stress and anxiety, potentially leading to sexual dysfunction.

- Vaginismus: Stress and anxiety play a role in vaginismus, and the vagus nerve is involved in regulating both. Vagal dysfunction could worsen anxiety and stress, indirectly contributing to vaginismus.

- Menopausal Symptoms: The vagus nerve's role in regulating stress and inflammation can impact symptoms like hot flashes and mood swings. Vagal dysfunction could exacerbate stress and inflammation, thereby potentially worsening menopausal symptoms.

Note that these conditions can have multiple causes, and vagus nerve dysfunction should not be seen as the sole factor. For accurate diagnosis and targeted treatment, consultation with healthcare professionals is essential.

In summary, while the vagus nerve doesn't have a pronounced direct influence on the female reproductive organs like it does on some other organs, its indirect roles in hormonal regulation, stress modulation, and autonomic balance can still have implications for female reproductive health. If you need more detailed information on any specific topic, consulting a gynecological textbook or related research articles would be beneficial.

References

1. Purves, D., Augustine, G., Fitzpatrick, D., Hall, W., LaMantia, A., Mooney, R., Platt, M. and White, L. (eds.), 2017. Neuroscience: 6th Edition. Oxford University Press USA.

2. Squire, L., Berg, D., Bloom, F.E., du Lac, S., Ghosh, A. and Spitzer, N.C. (eds.), 2012. Fundamental Neuroscience. 4th ed. Elsevier.

3. Llewellyn-Smith, I. J. and Verberne, A. J. M. (eds.) 2011. Central Regulation of Autonomic Functions, 2nd edn. Oxford University Press.

Chapter 21
The Vagus Nerve and The Brain

The vagus nerve plays a pivotal role in the function of the brainstem and has connections to various regions within the brain. Given the multifaceted nature of the vagus nerve and its extensive functions, understanding its interactions within the brainstem and broader brain structures is critical.

Vagus Nerve in the Brainstem:

The vagus nerve originates in the medulla oblongata, a portion of the brainstem. It includes the previously mentioned Dorsal Motor Nucleus, Nucleus Ambiguus, Solitary Nucleus (Nucleus of the Solitary Tract) and the Spinal Trigeminal Nucleus.

The vagus nerve interfaces with the reticular formation, a set of interconnected nuclei that play roles in sleep-wake cycles, alertness, and overall consciousness. It also has reciprocal connections with other cranial nerve nuclei in the brainstem, facilitating coordinated actions (e.g., the coordination of swallowing).

Vagus Nerve in the Broader Brain:

The vagus nerve sends sensory information, via the solitary tract nucleus, to the thalamus, which then relays it to various parts of the cortex. This pathway allows the brain to be aware of and respond to visceral sensations.

The vagus nerve has indirect connections with the hypothalamus. The hypothalamus, as a central autonomic center, interfaces with the vagus to regulate energy balance, stress responses, and other homeostatic functions.

The amygdala, involved in emotional responses, receives visceral sensory input from the vagus nerve. Such connections help explain why gut feelings or visceral sensations can influence our emotions.

The vagus communicates with the forebrain, which can modulate higher-level functions based on visceral feedback. For example, feeling "butterflies" in the stomach when nervous can affect cognitive processes in the forebrain.

Brain-Gut Axis

This concept underscores the bidirectional communication between the CNS and the gastrointestinal tract. The vagus nerve plays a key role in this, helping the brain monitor and respond to gut health, gut flora, and other gastrointestinal factors.

Brain-Related Conditions with Potential Links to Vagus Nerve Dysfunction:
- Anxiety Disorders: The vagus nerve regulates stress and relaxation responses, impacting the release of neurotransmitters. Reduced vagal tone could result in heightened stress responses, thereby contributing to anxiety disorders.
- Depression: Vagal nerve activity has been linked to mood regulation and activity in the dopamine and serotonin systems of the brain. Dysfunctional vagal activity could disrupt these pathways, particularly in the default mode network, contributing to depressive symptoms.
- Post-Traumatic Stress Disorder (PTSD): The vagus nerve is involved in the body's stress responses and emotional regulation. Poor vagal tone may result in an ineffective stress response, potentially contributing to PTSD symptoms.
- Migraines: The vagus nerve's role in inflammation and blood vessel dilation could affect migraines. Vagal dysfunction could exacerbate inflammatory pathways, thereby triggering or worsening migraines.
- Alzheimer's Disease: The vagus nerve has a role in inflammation, which is an area of concern in Alzheimer's pathology. Reduced vagal

activity could contribute to chronic inflammation, a known risk factor for Alzheimer's.

- Attention-Deficit/Hyperactivity Disorder (ADHD): The vagus nerve contributes to attention and impulse control through its regulatory effects on neurotransmitter release. Dysfunction in vagal tone could potentially exacerbate symptoms of ADHD by affecting neurotransmitter balance.

- Autism Spectrum Disorder: The vagus nerve is crucial for social bonding and emotional regulation, areas often affected in autism. Vagal dysfunction could potentially impact emotional and social development, contributing to autism symptoms.

- Sleep Disorders: The vagus nerve helps regulate circadian rhythms through its impact on stress hormones and relaxation. Disruptions in vagal activity could result in sleep disorders by affecting the sleep-wake cycle.

- Epilepsy: Vagus nerve stimulation is a treatment for certain types of epilepsy, suggesting a relationship between vagal activity and seizure control. Reduced or irregular vagal activity may contribute to dysregulated neural activity, potentially impacting epilepsy.

- Chronic Fatigue Syndrome: The vagus nerve plays a role in energy balance and homeostasis. Vagal dysfunction could contribute to systemic imbalances in energy, potentially leading to chronic fatigue.

These conditions can have multiple etiologies, and vagus nerve dysfunction should not be seen as the sole cause. For accurate diagnosis and treatment, consultation with healthcare professionals is essential.

The intricate interplay between the vagus nerve and the brain unveils the profound complexities of the human nervous system. Originating in the brainstem, the vagus nerve's extensive network not only bridges the cognitive realm with pivotal organs but also holds the potential to shape our emotional and physiological responses. Its influence, spanning from basic visceral sensations to intricate emotional reactions, underscores its significance in maintaining our body's equilibrium. Moreover, its association with various neurological and psychological conditions emphasizes the necessity of understanding its multifaceted roles. As modern medicine and neuroscience continue to advance, the vagus nerve stands out as a promising frontier, offering potential pathways to novel therapeutic interventions and a deeper comprehension of human well-being.

References

1. Breit, S., Kupferberg, A., Rogler, G. and Hasler, G., 2018. Vagus Nerve as Modulator of the Brain-Gut Axis in Psychiatric and Inflammatory Disorders. Front Psychiatry, 9, p.44. doi:10.3389/fpsyt.2018.00044. PMID: 29593576; PMCID: PMC5859128.

2. Purves, D., Augustine, G., Fitzpatrick, D., Hall, W., LaMantia, A., Mooney, R., Platt, M. and White, L. (eds.), 2017. Neuroscience: 6th Edition. Oxford University Press USA.

3. Squire, L., Berg, D., Bloom, F.E., du Lac, S., Ghosh, A. and Spitzer, N.C. (eds.), 2012. Fundamental Neuroscience. 4th ed. Elsevier.

4. Llewellyn-Smith, I.J. and Verberne, A.J.M. (eds.), 2011. Central Regulation of Autonomic Functions. 2nd ed. Oxford University Press.

5. Cryan, J.F., O'Riordan, K.J., Cowan, C.S.M., Sandhu, K.V., Bastiaanssen, T.F.S., Boehme, M., Codagnone, M.G., Cussotto, S., Fulling, C., Golubeva, A.V., Guzzetta, K.E., Jaggar, M., Long-Smith, C.M., Lyte, J.M., Martin, J.A., Molinero-Perez, A., Moloney, G., Morelli, E., Morillas, E., O'Connor, R., Cruz-Pereira, J.S., Peterson, V.L., Rea, K., Ritz, N.L., Sherwin, E., Spichak, S., Teichman, E.M., van de Wouw, M., Ventura-Silva, A.P., Wallace-Fitzsimons, S.E., Hyland, N., Clarke, G. and Dinan, T.G., 2019. The Microbiota-Gut-Brain Axis. Physiol Rev, 99(4), pp.1877-2013. doi:10.1152/physrev.00018.2018. PMID: 31460832.

6. Zhang, Y., Huang, Y., Li, H., Yan, Z., Zhang, Y., Liu, X., Hou, X., Chen, W., Tu, Y., Hodges, S., Chen, H., Liu, B. and Kong, J., 2021. Transcutaneous auricular vagus nerve stimulation (taVNS) for migraine: an fMRI study. Reg Anesth Pain Med, 46(2), pp.145-150. doi:10.1136/rapm-2020-102088. Epub 2020 Dec 1. PMID: 33262253.

Chapter 22
The Cholinergic Anti-Inflammatory Pathway of the Vagus Nerve

The cholinergic anti-inflammatory pathway (CAP) of the vagus nerve showcases the sophisticated interplay between the nervous system and the immune response. As a vital component of the body's parasympathetic division, this pathway stands at the crossroads of neuroimmunology. For clinicians, grasping the nuances of the CAP is paramount when considering the potential of the vagus nerve in regulating inflammation.

Overview of the Cholinergic Anti-Inflammatory Pathway:

The CAP epitomizes an advanced neural circuit. Primarily driven by efferent vagus nerve signaling, it possesses the power to reduce the production of pro-inflammatory cytokines, thereby attenuating the intensity of inflammatory reactions. The name "cholinergic" is derived from acetylcholine, the primary neurotransmitter of the vagus nerve, central to the anti-inflammatory cascade.

Diving deeper, the incoming signals from the vagus nerve detect inflammatory agents, transmitting this information to the brainstem. From there, a response is initiated and relayed through the outgoing vagus nerve, which then communicates with the splenic nerve. This culminates in the release of noradrenaline (NA) within the spleen. CD4+ T cells, equipped with the beta-2 adrenaline receptor (β2AR), absorb NA and subsequently produce acetylcholine (ACh). When ACh interacts with macrophages that have the α7 Nicotinic Acetylcholine Receptor (α7nAChR), it suppresses the release of proinflammatory cytokines (see image).

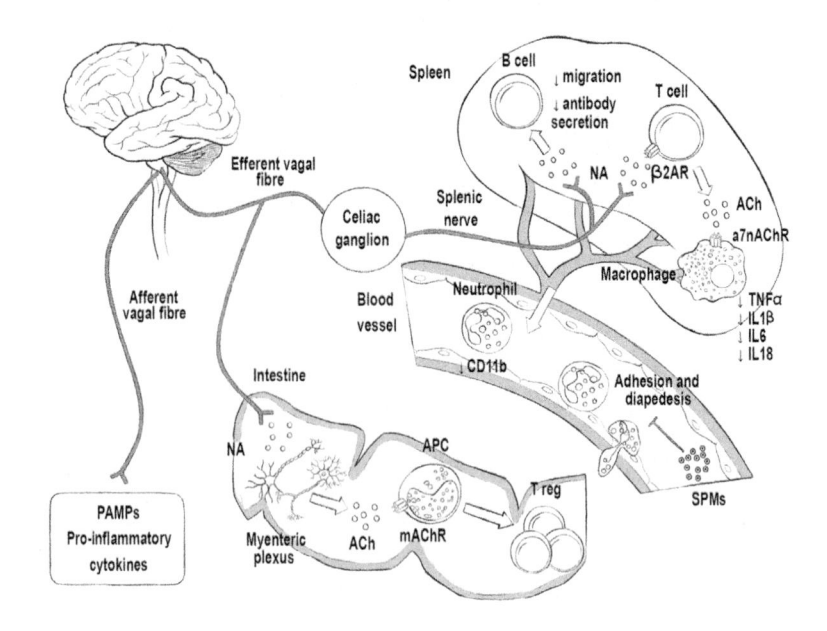

Moreover, in the realm of clinical relevance, the CAP has vast implications. Disorders or interruptions in this pathway can exacerbate diseases like sepsis, where uncontrolled inflammation can have fatal consequences. Conversely, targeted stimulation of this pathway unveils therapeutic potential. Clinical studies suggest that vagus nerve stimulation can significantly alleviate symptoms linked with rheumatoid arthritis and other inflammatory-rooted conditions like Inflammatory Bowel Disease (IBD).

As science continues to probe the complexities of the CAP, it remains a captivating domain in neuroimmunology. By enhancing our understanding, we stand to discover new therapeutic strategies, especially for conditions marked by rampant inflammation.

In summation, the cholinergic anti-inflammatory pathway offers a compelling synthesis of neuroscience and immunology concepts. It epitomizes the body's inherent capability to regulate inflammation. As research progresses, the possibility of groundbreaking treatments for inflammatory maladies becomes increasingly tangible.

References

1. Bonaz, B., Sinniger, V. and Pellissier, S., 2017. The Vagus Nerve in the Neuro-Immune Axis: Implications in the Pathology of the Gastrointestinal Tract. Front Immunol, 8, p.1452. doi:10.3389/fimmu.2017.01452. PMID: 29163522; PMCID: PMC5673632.

2. Wei, Y., Wang, T., Liao, L., Fan, X., Chang, L. and Hashimoto, K., 2022. Brain-spleen axis in health and diseases: A review and future perspective. Brain Res Bull, 182, pp.130-140. doi:10.1016/j.brainresbull.2022.02.008. Epub 2022 Feb 12. PMID: 35157987.

3. Simon, T., Kirk, J., Dolezalova, N., Guyot, M., Panzolini, C., Bondue, A., Lavergne, J., Hugues, S., Hypolite, N., Saeb-Parsy, K., Perkins, J., Macia, E., Sridhar, A., Vervoordeldonk, M.J., Glaichenhaus, N., Donegá, M. and Blancou, P., 2023. The cholinergic anti-inflammatory pathway inhibits inflammation without lymphocyte relay. Front Neurosci, 17, p.1125492. doi:10.3389/fnins.2023.1125492. PMID: 37123375; PMCID: PMC10140439.

4. Tracey, K.J., 2002. The inflammatory reflex. Nature, 420(6917), pp.853–859.

5. Pavlov, V.A. and Tracey, K.J., 2012. The vagus nerve and the inflammatory reflex—linking immunity and metabolism. Nature Reviews Endocrinology, 8(12), pp.743–754.

6. Ramos-Martínez, I.E., Rodríguez, M.C., Cerbón, M., Ramos-Martínez, J.C. and Ramos-Martínez, E.G., 2021. Role of the Cholinergic Anti-Inflammatory Reflex in Central Nervous System Diseases. *Int J Mol Sci*, 22(24), p.13427.

7. Koopman, F.A. et al., 2016. Vagus nerve stimulation inhibits cytokine production and attenuates disease severity in rheumatoid arthritis. Proceedings of the National Academy of Sciences, 113(29), pp.8284–8289.

Chapter 23
Vagus Nerve Dysfunction

Within the intricate network of our nervous system, the vagus nerve emerges as an essential player, bridging the brainstem to vital organs like the heart, lungs, and digestive tract. As the longest cranial nerve, its influence extends over a myriad physiological functions. However, its function isn't always consistent; its activity can manifest as low or high vagal tone, with each presenting its unique set of implications. Additionally, there's the phenomenon of excessive vagal tone, which can have significant repercussions on health. In this chapter, we will navigate the complexities of these vagal tone variations, exploring their causes, characteristics, and the broader effects on the body's symphony of functions.

Low Vagal Tone

A lowered functioning or decreased vagal tone can lead to a range of physiological, emotional, and psychological changes. Here is an exhaustive list of potential presentations of a patient with diminished vagus nerve function:

Physiological Symptoms and Signs
- Tachycardia: An increased resting heart rate due to reduced parasympathetic (vagal) control.
- Reduced Heart Rate Variability (HRV): HRV refers to the variation in the time interval between heartbeats. Lower HRV is often seen in conditions with diminished vagal tone and is associated with increased cardiovascular risk
- Dyspepsia: Problems in digestion due to reduced gut motility.

- Gastroesophageal Reflux Disease (GERD): Reduced vagal tone can impair the lower esophageal sphincter's function, leading to reflux.
- Constipation: Due to decreased gut motility.
- Reduced Gut Secretions: Diminished production of digestive enzymes and gastric juices.
- Shallow Breathing: Less diaphragmatic and deep breathing, potentially leading to lower oxygen saturation.
- Elevated Respiration: Higher respiratory rate may indicate low vagal tone or high sympathetic tone.

Emotional and Psychological Symptoms:
- Depression: Reduced vagal tone has been associated with depressive symptoms.
- Anxiety: Reduced parasympathetic activity can lead to heightened arousal states and anxiety.
- Difficulty in Emotional Regulation: Individuals may have challenges processing and regulating their emotions.
- Reduced Social Bonding: The vagus nerve is believed to play a role in creating feelings of connection and social bonding. Reduced function can lead to feelings of social disconnection.
- Decreased Resilience to Stress: Reduced capacity to cope with and recover from stressors.

Cognitive Symptoms:
- Attentional Problems: Difficulties in maintaining attention and being easily distracted.
- Memory Issues: Potential challenges in memory retrieval and formation.

Other Potential Signs and Symptoms:
- Reduced Anti-inflammatory Reflex: The vagus nerve plays a role in modulating inflammation. Reduced function can result in heightened inflammatory responses.

- Fatigue: General feelings of tiredness and lack of energy.
- Weakened Immune System: Leading to an increased susceptibility to infections.
- Difficulty in Swallowing: Due to reduced muscular control in the esophagus.
- Voice Changes: Potential hoarseness or changes in voice quality because the vagus nerve also innervates the larynx.

Potential Behavioral Symptoms:
- Reduced Gag Reflex: The gag reflex can be diminished or absent.
- Difficulty Reading Facial Expressions: Challenges in recognizing and interpreting others' emotional facial cues.

It's important to note that many of these symptoms are nonspecific and can be associated with a variety of medical and psychological conditions. Therefore, a comprehensive assessment by a healthcare professional is crucial to determine the root cause and appropriate intervention. Furthermore, some individuals might have a naturally lower vagal tone without presenting any of the aforementioned symptoms. The implications of vagal tone can vary from person to person, and many factors, including genetics, environment, and individual experiences, influence its manifestation.

Excessive Vagal Tone

Excessive vagal tone, or hyperactivity of the vagus nerve, can manifest with a variety of symptoms. Here's an exhaustive list and description of potential presentations in a patient with increased vagal function:

Physiological Symptoms and Signs

- Bradycardia: A slower-than-normal heart rate.
- Hypotension: Reduced blood pressure, particularly upon standing (orthostatic hypotension).
- Syncope: Fainting or sudden, temporary loss of consciousness often due to a drop in blood flow to the brain. This can be triggered by

a variety of stimuli, like sudden emotional distress.

- Hyperactive Bowel Sounds: Increased gut motility can lead to more noticeable bowel sounds.
- Diarrhea: Increased peristalsis and gut motility can lead to frequent bowel movements.
- Stomach Cramping: Due to hyperactivity of the digestive tract muscles.
- Bradypnea: Abnormally slow breathing rate.
- Dyspnea: Difficulty breathing.

Emotional and Psychological Symptoms:

- Calmness or Excessive Relaxation: While a balanced vagal tone is associated with a calm demeanor, excessive vagal tone might make an individual overly calm or relaxed, potentially to the point of apathy.
- Reduced Stress Response: While decreased stress response might seem beneficial, it could be detrimental in situations that require prompt and alert reactions.

Cognitive Symptoms:

- Potential Cognitive Lethargy: Overly calm states might make individuals less reactive or slow to process information.

Other Potential Signs and Symptoms:

- Excessive Salivation: The vagus nerve influences salivary gland secretion.
- Difficulty Swallowing: Dysphagia might occur due to altered muscular coordination.

Potential Behavioral Symptoms:

- Enhanced Gag Reflex: Increased sensitivity can lead to easy triggering of the gag reflex.

Specific Reflex Responses:

- Vasovagal Syncope: This is a specific response where certain triggers (e.g., the sight of blood, intense emotional distress) can lead to a sudden drop in heart rate and blood pressure, resulting in fainting.

Potential Complications in Medical Settings:

- Increased Risk during Intubation: Excessive vagal stimulation during procedures like intubation can lead to bradycardia or even cardiac arrest in susceptible individuals.

Again, it's crucial to recognize that these manifestations can be present in various conditions unrelated to vagal tone. Therefore, a thorough assessment by a healthcare professional is essential. In some settings, increased vagal tone might be beneficial (e.g., for certain anxiety disorders), but excessive vagal activity can be problematic in other situations.

References

1. Purves, D., Augustine, G., Fitzpatrick, D., Hall, W., LaMantia, A., Mooney, R., Platt, M. and White, L. (eds.), 2017. Neuroscience: 6th Edition. Oxford University Press USA.

2. Squire, L., Berg, D., Bloom, F.E., du Lac, S., Ghosh, A. and Spitzer, N.C. (eds.), 2012. Fundamental Neuroscience. 4th ed. Elsevier.

3. Llewellyn-Smith, I.J. and Verberne, A.J.M. (eds.), 2011. Central Regulation of Autonomic Functions. 2nd ed. Oxford University Press.

4. Bonaz, B., Sinniger, V. and Pellissier, S., 2016. Vagal tone: effects on sensitivity, motility, and inflammation. Neurogastroenterol Motil, 28(4), pp.455-462. doi:10.1111/nmo.12817. PMID: 27010234.

5. McLaughlin, K.A., Rith-Najarian, L., Dirks, M.A. and Sheridan, M.A., 2015. Low vagal tone magnifies the association between psychosocial stress exposure and internalizing psychopathology in adolescents. J Clin Child Adolesc Psychol, 44(2), pp.314-328. doi:10.1080/15374416.2013.843464. PMID: 24156380; PMCID: PMC4076387.

6. Hage, B., Britton, B., Daniels, D., Heilman, K., Porges, S.W. and Halaris, A., 2019. Low cardiac vagal tone index by heart rate variability differentiates bipolar from major depression. World J Biol Psychiatry, 20(5), pp.359-367. doi:10.1080/15622975.2017.1376113. PMID: 28895492.

7. Hausken, T., Svebak, S., Wilhelmsen, I., Haug, T.T., Olafsen, K., Pettersson, E., Hveem, K. and Berstad, A., 1993. Low vagal tone and antral dysmotility in patients with functional dyspepsia. Psychosom Med, 55(1), pp.12-22. doi:10.1097/00006842-199301000-00004. PMID: 8446737.

8. Weber, C.S., Thayer, J.F., Rudat, M., Wirtz, P.H., Zimmermann-Viehoff, F., Thomas, A., Perschel, F.H., Arck, P.C. and Deter, H.C., 2010. Low vagal tone is associated with impaired post stress recovery of cardiovascular, endocrine, and immune markers. Eur J Appl Physiol, 109(2), pp.201-211. doi:10.1007/s00421-009-1341-x. PMID: 20052593.

9. Thayer, J.F., Yamamoto, S.S. and Brosschot, J.F., 2010. The relationship of autonomic imbalance, heart rate variability and cardiovascular disease risk factors. Int J Cardiol, 141(2), pp.122-131. doi:10.1016/j.ijcard.2009.09.543. PMID: 19910061.

10. Kim, S.H., Lim, K.R., Seo, J.H., Ryu, D.R., Lee, B.K., Cho, B.R. and Chun, K.J., 2022. Higher heart rate variability as a predictor of atrial fibrillation in patients with hypertension. Sci Rep, 12(1), p.3702. doi:10.1038/s41598-022-07783-3. PMID: 35260686; PMCID: PMC8904557.

Chapter 24
Causes of Vagus Nerve Dysfunction

The vagus nerve, a key component of the body's autonomic nervous system, can be vulnerable to dysfunction due to a variety of causes. One of the primary culprits is compression, which can be either transient or constant, affecting the normal signaling processes of the nerve.

Physical trauma, particularly resulting from surgeries or injuries to the head and neck region, can directly damage or impede the nerve's function. Additionally, neurological disorders such as Multiple Sclerosis (MS) and Parkinson's disease can disrupt the normal operation of the vagus nerve.

Systemic conditions like diabetes can also play a role, given the disease's potential to induce neuropathy. Moreover, external factors like certain medications, chronic alcoholism, and exposure to toxins can contribute to vagus nerve dysfunction, further underscoring the complexity of factors influencing its health.

Compression Disorders

Compression of the vagus nerve can lead to a variety of clinical manifestations, including changes in vagal tone. However, the exact outcome — whether there's an increase (excessive) or decrease (reduced) in vagal tone — will largely depend on the nature, location, and intensity of the compression, as well as the affected fibers within the nerve. Here's how compression might influence vagal tone:

Nature of Compression:

Continuous vs. Intermittent: Constant compression may desensitize the nerve over time, leading to a reduced vagal tone, while intermittent compression might stimulate it, potentially increasing its tone.

Location of Compression:

Proximal vs. Distal Compression: Compression closer to the nerve's origin in the brainstem might have a more generalized effect on various functions of the vagus nerve, whereas compression at a more distal location might affect specific branch functions.

Intensity of Compression:

Mild vs. Severe Compression: Mild compression might act as a stimulant to the nerve, leading to increased vagal tone. In contrast, severe compression might impede the nerve's ability to conduct signals effectively, leading to reduced vagal tone.

Affected Fibers:

The vagus nerve comprises multiple fiber types, including motor (efferent) and sensory (afferent) fibers. Compression might not affect all these fibers uniformly. For instance, selective compression of efferent fibers might lead to reduced parasympathetic output and therefore decreased vagal tone. Conversely, stimulation of afferent fibers might induce reflexive increases in vagal tone.

Compensatory Mechanisms:

The body might compensate for chronic compression of the vagus nerve by modulating the tone of the nerve over time. For example, initial compression might lead to increased vagal tone (due to the stimulatory effect of the compression), but with time and continuous compression, the nerve might adapt, and vagal tone might normalize or even decrease.

Pathological Processes:

Tumors, Cysts, or Vascular Malformations: These can compress the vagus nerve. Depending on their growth rate, they might cause either increased or decreased vagal tone. Slow-growing masses might initially stimulate the nerve but can lead to decreased function over time as they exert more pressure.

CAUSES OF VAGUS NERVE DYSFUNCTION

External Factors:

Trauma or Surgical Interventions: Physical injury or surgical procedures near the path of the vagus nerve might compress it, either directly or due to resultant inflammation and swelling.

Reflex Mechanisms:

Compression might activate reflex pathways that modulate vagal activity. For instance, afferent fibers might convey sensory information to the central nervous system upon compression, triggering reflexive changes in vagal tone.

Potential Sites of Compression of the Vagus Nerve

Jugular Foramen: The vagus nerve exits the skull through this foramen.

- Possible Causes: Cervical instability, tumors, bone abnormalities, lymphadenopathy or inflammation around this region can compress the nerve.

Carotid Sheath: The vagus nerve descends within the carotid sheath alongside the carotid artery and internal jugular vein.

- Possible Causes: Segmental cervical instability, lymphadenopathy, bony abnormalities like spurs, any mass within the sheath, such as a carotid artery aneurysm, goiter or tumors.

Mediastinum: The vagus nerve has branches in the mediastinum, particularly the recurrent laryngeal nerves.

- Possible Causes: Lung cancer, aortic aneurysm, or other mediastinal masses can compress branches of the vagus here.

Anterior to Subclavian Artery: The right recurrent laryngeal nerve hooks around the right subclavian artery.

- Possible Causes: Aneurysms or other vascular abnormalities of the subclavian artery.

Aortic Arch: The left recurrent laryngeal nerve hooks around the aortic arch.

THE VAGUS NERVE

Possible Causes: Aortic aneurysms or dilation.

Esophageal Hiatus of the Diaphragm: The vagus nerve passes through the esophageal hiatus to enter the abdomen.

- Possible Causes: Hiatal hernias can compress the nerve here.

Within the Abdomen: After passing through the diaphragm, the vagus nerve supplies branches to the abdominal organs.

- Possible Causes: Abdominal aortic aneurysms or tumors within the abdomen. Accidental compression or damage during surgeries.

Potential Causes of Cervical Segmental Instability:
- Ehlers-Danlos Syndrome (EDS): A hereditary connective tissue disorder causing hypermobility and laxity in the joints. Individuals with EDS often have weakened connective tissue, which can lead to instability in various joints, including those in the cervical spine.
- Trauma: Acute injuries such as whiplash from motor vehicle accidents or sports injuries can damage the ligaments and other stabilizing structures in the neck, leading to instability.
- Rheumatoid Arthritis: An autoimmune disease that can cause destruction of the joints, potentially leading to instability, especially in the cervical region.
- Osteoarthritis: Degeneration of the cervical joints and discs over time can lead to instability, especially if there is a loss of disc height.
- Congenital Anomalies: Some individuals may be born with structural abnormalities in the cervical spine that predispose them to instability.
- Surgical Complications: Certain neck surgeries, especially those that involve fusion or removal of stabilizing structures, can result in instability if the fusion doesn't heal properly or if the hardware fails.
- Infections: Infections such as osteomyelitis can erode cervical vertebrae and the intervening discs, leading to potential instability.
- Tumors: Neoplastic growth, either primary or metastatic, can erode

or displace cervical spine structures, causing instability.

- Degenerative Disc Disease: A condition where the cervical discs become dehydrated and lose height, potentially leading to instability.
- Neuromuscular Conditions: Conditions such as cerebral palsy or muscular dystrophy may lead to muscle imbalances or weaknesses that can contribute to cervical instability.

It's crucial to recognize that while this list encompasses many potential causes of cervical segmental instability, the clinical presentation and severity can vary widely based on the underlying cause. Any suspicions of cervical instability should warrant a thorough evaluation by a medical professional.

In clinical practice, it's essential to determine the cause of the compression and its exact impact on the vagus nerve. Compression might lead to a mix of symptoms, including those not directly related to changes in vagal tone. An accurate diagnosis requires a thorough examination, and potential imaging studies like MRI or CT scans, to understand the nature and extent of the compression.

Upper Jugular Lymphadenopathy and Its Impact on the Vagus Nerve

Lymphadenopathy refers to the enlargement of one or more lymph nodes, typically resulting from infection, inflammation, or malignancy. The upper jugular lymph nodes, situated adjacent to the jugular vein in the neck, play a crucial role in draining lymph from the pharynx, posterior part of the nasal cavity, and tonsils. When these nodes become enlarged, they can pose compressive risks to neighboring anatomical structures, including the vagus nerve.

Lymphadenopathy and Vagal Compression

Positional Relationship: The vagus nerve's proximity to the upper jugular lymph nodes means that any enlargement or inflammation of these nodes can lead to compression of the nerve as it traverses through the jugular foramen.

Compression Symptoms: Symptoms may reflect high or low vagal tone, look at sections on each to determine what type.

Pathological Causes: While infections are a common cause for transient lymphadenopathy, other causes, including malignancies like lymphomas or metastatic cancers, can also lead to persistent swelling of the upper jugular lymph nodes. The chronic nature of such swellings poses a longer-term risk for vagus nerve compression.

Vagus nerve dysfunction can stem from a myriad of causes, ranging from compression syndromes and neuropathies to trauma and neurodegenerative diseases. Additionally, external factors such as certain medications, alcoholism, and exposure to toxins can further compromise its function. Given the intricacies of the vagus nerve and its pivotal role in numerous bodily functions, it's crucial for individuals experiencing potential symptoms to consult with a clinician trained in vagus nerve examination. Their expertise ensures a comprehensive understanding of the nerve's involvement in a patient's condition and facilitates accurate diagnosis and management.

References

1. Purves, D., Augustine, G., Fitzpatrick, D., Hall, W., LaMantia, A., Mooney, R., Platt, M. and White, L. (eds.), 2017. Neuroscience: 6th Edition. Oxford University Press USA.

2. Squire, L., Berg, D., Bloom, F.E., du Lac, S., Ghosh, A. and Spitzer, N.C. (eds.), 2012. Fundamental Neuroscience. 4th ed. Elsevier.

3. Llewellyn-Smith, I. J. and Verberne, A. J. M. (eds.) 2011. Central Regulation of Autonomic Functions, 2nd edn. Oxford University Press.

Chapter 25
Vagus Nerve Assessment

Clinical examinations of the vagus nerve are designed to assess its integrity and function, which are vital for various physiological processes. Through these examinations, clinicians can deduce whether a person has high, low, or excessive vagal activity or tone.

Initial Testing Procedure

1. Palate Elevation and Gag Reflex: This test checks the movement of the soft palate and the uvula when a patient says "ahh". The gag reflex is also tested by touching the back of the throat with a tongue depressor. Abnormalities here, such as a leaning uvula or a reduced gag reflex, can hint at vagus nerve dysfunction, as this nerve controls the muscles of the soft palate (see image).

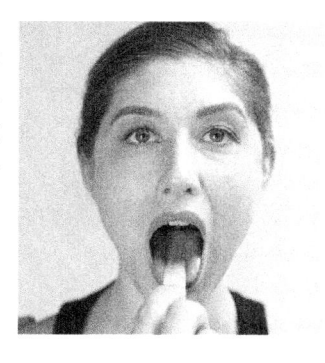

2. Voice Assessment: The patient's voice is analyzed for any unusual nasal quality or hoarseness. Since the vagus nerve innervates a majority of the larynx muscles, any voice changes can be indicative of nerve dysfunction.

3. Swallowing Test: The patient is asked to swallow water. If they cough, choke, or struggle, it can suggest an issue with the vagus nerve, which plays a role in swallowing.

4. Cough Reflex: This involves asking the patient to cough. A weakened

THE VAGUS NERVE

reflex might suggest vagal dysfunction as the cough reflex is largely mediated by the vagus nerve.

5. Heart Rate Monitoring: The vagus nerve plays a role in modulating heart rate. Thus, an unusually high or low resting heart rate might indicate a change in vagal tone (see image).

6. Observing Respiratory Patterns: A change in breathing rate and appearance could be related to a change in vagus nerve function (see image).

7. Assessment of Organ Function: Symptoms related to the stomach, intestines, and other organs can hint at vagal dysfunction, as the vagus nerve affects their operation.

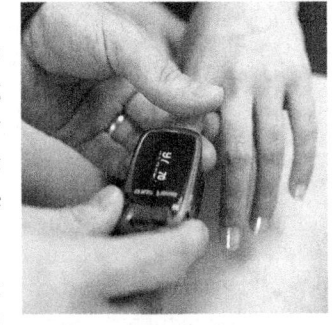

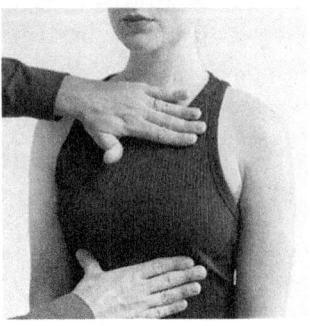

8. Examination of the External Ear: Testing the skin sensitivity in the concha region of the ear can provide insights into the function of the auricular vagus nerve.

Neurodynamic Assessment

By palpating the carotid sheath in the neck, where the vagus nerve is located, any potential tension or tenderness can be identified during cervical spine active range of motion. Although the vagus nerve itself cannot be distinctly felt as it's deeply encased, clinicians can sense its pathway and infer its condition based on the tissue tension and the patient's reported sensations (see image).

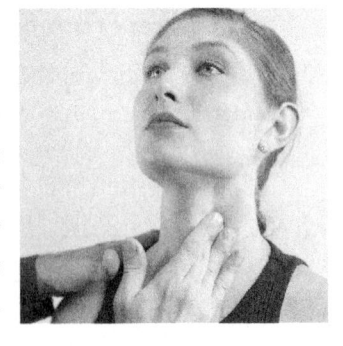

Heart Rate Variability (HRV)

HRV, or Heart Rate Variability, is a measure of the variability or fluctuations in the time intervals between consecutive heartbeats. These intervals are often referred to as inter-beat intervals or RR intervals, where "R" is a point denoting the peak of the QRS complex in the heart's electrical cycle.

Understanding RR Intervals

The heart doesn't beat in a fixed rhythm as one might intuitively think. Instead, there are slight variations in the time between each heartbeat. This is especially evident when you consider that the heart needs to constantly adapt to the demands of the body, whether we're resting, exercising, or experiencing emotional stress.

High vs Low HRV

High HRV generally indicates healthy vagal (parasympathetic) activity. Conversely, low HRV suggests low vagus nerve activity or high sympathetic activity. Sometimes a person may have excessive vagal tone expressed as high HRV, but will have symptoms such as bradycardia, slow or difficult breathing and fatigue.

Gold Standard Methods of Measuring HRV

Electrocardiogram (ECG or EKG): An ECG records the electrical activity of the heart. It provides precise and detailed information about the intervals between heartbeats, making it the gold standard for measuring HRV. HRV metrics are often derived from a 24-hour Holter monitor, a portable ECG device.

Clinic or At-Home Methods

- Heart Rate Chest Straps: Devices like the Polar H10 strap can measure beat-to-beat intervals, providing accurate HRV data. They use electrical signals, much like an ECG, but are more comfortable and less cumbersome.

- Photoplethysmography (PPG): Devices like wrist-worn fitness trackers and some smartphone apps use PPG to measure heart rate. PPG measures blood volume changes in the microvasculature of tissue (like the fingertip or earlobe) using a light source and a photodetector. While these devices can provide HRV metrics, they may be less accurate than ECG-based methods, especially during movement or poor perfusion.

- Dedicated HRV Apps: Some apps, like Elite HRV or HRV4Training, allow users to measure and track their HRV using either a compatible chest strap or the smartphone's built-in camera (though the latter might be less accurate).
- Finger Sensors: Some medical-grade devices, often used in clinics, use sensors that can be attached to the finger to measure HRV, offering a balance between accuracy and convenience.

While measuring HRV has become more accessible, interpreting the data requires some expertise. HRV is influenced by a wide range of factors, including:

- Age (HRV generally decreases with age)

- Fitness level (more fit individuals often have higher HRV)

- Stress (both acute and chronic stress can reduce HRV)

- Sleep quality and duration

- Alcohol or caffeine consumption

- Illness or infection

Because of these variables, it's essential to interpret HRV in the context of individual baseline values and not just absolute numbers. It's also beneficial to track HRV over time rather than making decisions based on a single reading.

In clinical and research settings, HRV is sometimes used as a biomarker for conditions like cardiovascular diseases, mental health disorders, and even predicting surgical outcomes or recovery. In the general public and among athletes, HRV is becoming a popular metric for assessing stress, recovery, and overall health.

References

1. Purves, D., Augustine, G., Fitzpatrick, D., Hall, W., LaMantia, A., Mooney, R., Platt, M. and White, L. (eds.), 2017. Neuroscience: 6th Edition. Oxford University Press USA.

2. Squire, L., Berg, D., Bloom, F.E., du Lac, S., Ghosh, A. and Spitzer, N.C. (eds.), 2012. Fundamental Neuroscience. 4th ed. Elsevier.

3. Llewellyn-Smith, I.J. and Verberne, A.J.M. (eds.), 2011. Central Regulation of Autonomic Functions. 2nd ed. Oxford University Press.

4. Taylor, A., Mourad, F., Kerry, R. and Hutting, N., 2021. A guide to cranial nerve testing for musculoskeletal clinicians. J Man Manip Ther, 29(6), pp.376-389. doi:10.1080/10669817.2021.1937813. PMID: 34182898; PMCID: PMC8725776.

5. Shahrokhi, M. and Asuncion, R.M.D., 2023. Neurologic Exam. In: StatPearls [Internet]. Treasure Island, FL: StatPearls Publishing; 2023 Jan. PMID: 32491521.

6. Tiwari, R., Kumar, R., Malik, S., Raj, T. and Kumar, P., 2021. Analysis of Heart Rate Variability and Implication of Different Factors on Heart Rate Variability. Curr Cardiol Rev, 17(5). doi:10.2174/1573403X16999201231203854. PMID: 33390146; PMCID: PMC8950456.

Chapter 26
Treatment of the Vagus Nerve

To address issues related to vagus nerve dysfunction, it's essential to target the compression of the vagus nerve, which often occurs near the jugular foramen or within the carotid sheath. While the root cause can vary—ranging from localized tumors and swollen lymph nodes to structural abnormalities of the bone—many individuals find relief through direct manipulation of the nerve and neurodynamic techniques. A cornerstone of effective treatment also involves stabilizing the cervical spine, primarily through targeted strengthening exercises. Finally, vagus nerve stimulation can be achieved either through a range of at-home techniques or via transcutaneous auricular vagus nerve stimulation. This chapter will delve into these various treatment approaches.

In this book, I'll provide an overview of various techniques that are best administered by trained clinicians. Remember, the content herein is purely informational. Methods to mobilize the vagus nerve, particularly as it departs from the jugular foramen and moves through the carotid sheath, have consistently benefited many of my patients. Additionally, therapies such as photobiomodulation can be employed to enhance the outcomes. A pivotal component in this process often lies in strengthening the cervical musculature. Intriguingly, a significant number of individuals with vagus nerve issues also exhibit some form of cervical weakness. Strengthening exercises have, in many cases, ameliorated their symptoms, though the exact reason remains a subject of ongoing research.

My goal is to equip as many clinicians as possible with these methodologies. In doing so, I hope to provide patients globally with interventions that tackle the root cause of their vagus nerve dysfunction, as opposed to merely offering temporary relief through electrical or basic at-home stimulations.

Direct Nerve Manipulation

Direct manipulation techniques, which focus on specific sections of the nerve and its branches, have shown promising therapeutic benefits. For instance, techniques that guide the vagus nerve within the carotid sheath can alleviate restrictions and enhance the nerve's mobility. Similarly, maneuvers that address the recurrent laryngeal nerve aim to improve issues tied to vocal cord functionality. The intent of these practices is not just to alleviate symptoms but to target potential root causes, such as compressions or restrictions that hinder nerve function. As with any intricate medical procedure, precision, comprehensive knowledge of the anatomy, and a patient-centric approach are paramount. These techniques, when executed correctly, present a valuable repertoire for clinicians aiming to harness the therapeutic capabilities of the vagus nerve while ensuring patient safety and comfort.

Transcutaneous Auricular Vagus Nerve Stimulation (taVNS)

Transcutaneous auricular vagus nerve stimulation (taVNS) is a cutting-edge, non-invasive approach to harnessing the vast potential of the vagus nerve to treat various medical conditions. By targeting the auricular branch of the vagus nerve, taVNS allows for the modulation of parasympathetic activity, thereby influencing a plethora of physiological systems. As the scientific and medical communities continue to explore the full range of the vagus nerve's effects, taVNS offers a promising, less invasive alternative to implanted vagus nerve stimulators, potentially transforming the therapeutic landscape for conditions ranging from mood disorders to chronic pain.

taVNS can be tailored to individual needs, considering factors like frequency, pulse width, and intensity. To gauge the effectiveness of taVNS, monitoring heart rate before and during stimulation is key. An effective session typically results in a reduction of heart rate by 3 to 4 beats per minute, aligning with respiratory sinus arrhythmia. In cases where there's little to no change, or if the heart rate remains within regular boundaries, the effectiveness of taVNS might be questioned. As such, taVNS should be viewed as one among various potential interventions for the vagus nerve. It might also be integrated into recovery plans for vagus nerve palsy, but always as part of a broader strategy.

taVNS is not suitable for everyone. It's advised against its use for those with active ear infections as stimulation might worsen them. Additionally, individuals who've recently undergone ear surgeries, have ear injuries, or have cochlear implants and other electronic devices like pacemakers are also advised to refrain from taVNS. Furthermore, individuals known to be hypersensitive to electrical stimulation should avoid the procedure due to potential adverse reactions.

Safety Research A meta-analysis was completed by Kim et al (2022) that examined adverse events (AEs) linked with taVNS. The study revealed a bias in reporting, with nearly 50% of studies not mentioning any AEs. They assumed no AEs were present in these studies. Their meta-analysis found no difference in the risk or intensity of AEs between active taVNS and controls. The most common AEs were ear pain, headache, and tingling, but none were severe. Thus, taVNS appears to be a safe treatment option.

Important Note on taVNS:

It's postulated that taVNS offers greater efficacy in individuals without vagus nerve compression. Compression can hinder effective transmission of electrical signals, thereby potentially reducing the therapeutic benefits of taVNS. Identifying and assessing for vagus nerve compression might be crucial in optimizing outcomes.

Bilateral vs. Unilateral Stimulation:

Unilateral Stimulation: Often preferred by some clinicians and researchers, typically involving the left ear to avoid potential cardiac effects linked to right-sided vagal stimulation, but this has been refuted by researchers.

Bilateral Stimulation: More and more are utilizing this method in research and clinically. Therapeutic effects are likely improved relative to one-sided stimulation.

Implanted Vagus Nerve Stimulators:

Implanted vagus nerve stimulators are medical devices designed to deliver electrical impulses directly to the vagus nerve, a major nerve running from the brainstem to the abdomen. Surgically implanted under the skin, typically in the chest region, these stimulators consist of a pulse generator and lead wires that attach to the vagus nerve in the neck. Once activated, they send controlled electrical signals to modulate nerve activity. Regular follow-ups and adjustments are necessary to ensure the stimulator functions effectively and safely for the patient.

Comparison to Implanted Vagus Nerve Stimulators:

taVNS provides a non-invasive option compared to surgically implanted devices. From a cost perspective, taVNS is generally more cost-effective. Although both approaches can result in side effects, the invasive methods come with added risks inherent to surgical procedures and the actual implant. Despite these risks, both have demonstrated effectiveness in managing several conditions. However, it's important to note that invasive vagus nerve stimulators, while advantageous for numerous patients, also come with their set of potential side effects.

- Voice changes or hoarseness: This is one of the most common side effects, given the proximity of the vagus nerve to the vocal cords.
- Cough or shortness of breath: Some patients might experience a cough or feel short of breath, especially when the device is stimulating the nerve.
- Difficulty swallowing: Stimulation might occasionally interfere with the act of swallowing.
- Tingling or pricking sensation in the skin: Some users describe a sensation similar to pins and needles.
- Neck pain: Discomfort or pain might be felt in the area where the device stimulates the nerve.

- Headaches: Some patients have reported headaches as a result of the stimulation.

- Difficulty sleeping: The device might interfere with regular sleeping patterns for some users.

- Nausea or vomiting: Rare, but some patients might feel nauseous or even vomit due to the stimulation.

- Heart palpitations: Some patients might feel an irregularity in their heartbeat.

- Worsening of seizure symptoms: For those using VNS for epilepsy, there's a slight risk that the seizures could become more frequent or more severe.

- Infection: As with any surgical procedure, there's a risk of infection at the implantation site.

It's crucial for patients to communicate with their healthcare providers about any side effects they're experiencing. Adjustments can often be made to the device's settings to mitigate some of these issues.

Disclaimer: This chapter provides an informative overview of taVNS. It doesn't promote or guarantee its effectiveness for specific individuals. Clinicians should be equipped with proper training and adhere to regional licensing and legal guidelines. Patients should always seek taVNS under the guidance of qualified professionals.

In conclusion, while many individuals experience significant improvement through in-person treatments such as direct nerve manipulation and taVNS, it's essential to note that a considerable number can also benefit from the techniques we'll introduce in the next chapter. These self-help methods serve as an accessible and effective approach for those who might not have immediate access to more direct interventions.

References

1. Bonaz, B., Sinniger, V., Hoffmann, D., Clarençon, D., Mathieu, N. & Dantzer, C., 2016. Chronic vagus nerve stimulation in Crohn's disease: a 6-month follow-up pilot study. *Neurogastroenterology & Motility*, 28(6), pp. 948-953.

2. He, W., Jing, X., Wang, X., Rong, P., Li, L., Shi, H., ... & Zhu, B., 2013. Transcutaneous auricular vagus nerve stimulation as a complementary therapy for pediatric epilepsy: a pilot trial. *Epilepsy & Behavior*, 28(3), pp. 343-346.

3. Kim, AY., Marduy, A., de Melo, PS., Gianlorenco, AC., Kim, CK., Choi, H., Song, JJ. & Fregni, F., 2022. Safety of transcutaneous auricular vagus nerve stimulation (taVNS): a systematic review and meta-analysis. *Sci Rep*, 12(1), p. 22055.

4. Peuker, E.T. & Filler, T.J., 2002. The nerve supply of the human auricle. *Clinical Anatomy*, 15(1), pp. 35-37.

5. Rong, P., Liu, J., Wang, L., Liu, R., Fang, J., Zhao, J., ... & Kong, J., 2016. Effect of transcutaneous auricular vagus nerve stimulation on major depressive disorder: A nonrandomized controlled pilot study. *Journal of Affective Disorders*, 195, pp. 172-179.

6. Yuan, H. & Silberstein, S.D., 2016. Vagus nerve stimulation and headache. *Headache: The Journal of Head and Face Pain*, 56(3), pp. 536-544.

Chapter 27
Optimising Vagal Tone

Navigating the myriad of treatment options for vagus nerve dysfunction can be challenging. Which methods truly make a difference? While definitive answers are still emerging, my belief is rooted in a fundamental principle: the vagus nerve can only operate effectively when its pathway is unobstructed. Addressing fascial restrictions, adhesions, and other compression sources is a preliminary step. Only after these obstructions are managed can we begin strengthening the cervical muscles, addressing any instability that might contribute to compression through muscle guarding. Finally, taVNS can be introduced to rejuvenate the nerve, either in tandem with or exclusively through at-home techniques.

Addressing Vagus Nerve Compression

To alleviate symptoms linked to vagus nerve dysfunction, a common approach involves focusing on where the nerve gets compressed, such as near the jugular foramen or inside the carotid sheath. This compression can arise from various sources like adhesions, fascial restrictions, muscular guarding, tumors, lymph nodes swelling, or bone abnormalities. Solutions range from directly handling the nerve, using neurodynamic techniques, to stabilizing the cervical spine. Furthermore, stimulating the vagus nerve can be done either with at-home methods and/or using transcutaneous auricular vagus nerve stimulation.

Augment Vagal Tone from Home: Cervical Spine Strengthening

Many individuals find relief through targeted neck strengthening exercises, focusing especially on the scalenes, sternocleidomastoid, and the deep neck flexor group. These specific muscles often lag in strength, contributing to overall neck instability. For those keen on exploring these exercises, it's advisable to seek guidance from a clinician certified in cervical spine rehabilitation.

One can initiate neck strengthening using simple methods, progressing to more advanced levels as strength and endurance improve. Here's a detailed guide to cervical spine strengthening across three levels of progression:

Level 1: Gravity-Assisted

At this initial stage, the weight of your head provides the resistance against which your neck muscles work.

Flexion Level 1:
1. Start by lying on your back with legs out straight or knees bent. Feet planted on the ground.
2. Lift your head off the floor or bed, look towards your feet.
3. Hold for 1-3 seconds and then relax.
4. Repeat 5 times, rest, then repeat up to 3 times. (see image)

Lateral Flexion Level 1:
1. Lie on your side.
2. Attempt to touch your ear to your shoulder without raising your shoulder.
3. Hold for 1-3 seconds and then relax.
4. Repeat 5 times, rest, then repeat up to 3 times. Make sure you do both

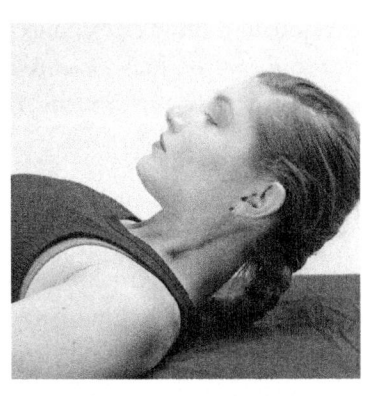

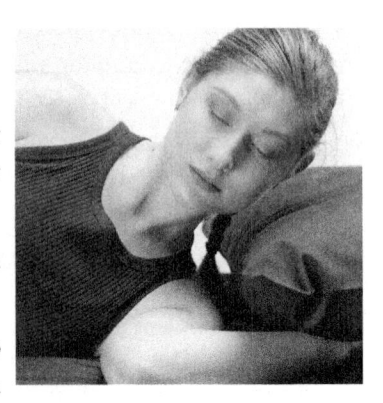

sides.

Flexion Level 2:
1. Start by lying on your back with legs out straight or knees bent. Feet planted on the ground.
2. Lift your head off the floor or bed, look towards your feet.
3. Hold for 10 seconds and then relax.
4. Repeat 5 times, rest, then repeat up to 3 times.
5. To make it harder, add hand pressure.

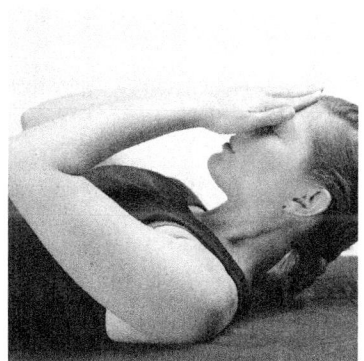

Lateral Flexion Level 2:
1. Lie on your side.
2. Attempt to touch your ear to your shoulder without raising your shoulder.
3. Hold for 10 seconds and then relax.
4. Repeat 5 times, rest, then repeat up to 3 times. Make sure you do both sides.

PLEASE NOTE: As with any exercise, ensure that movements are controlled and that you maintain proper alignment. If pain or discomfort is felt, it is crucial to reassess technique, reduce resistance, or consult a physical therapist or medical professional.

Augment Vagal Tone from Home: Breathing

1. Diaphragmatic Breathing (Abdominal or Belly Breathing)

Sit or lie down in a comfortable position. Place one hand on your chest and another on your abdomen. Breathe in slowly through the nose, allowing your abdomen to rise as you fill your lungs with air. Exhale slowly through your mouth or nose. The hand on your abdomen should move more than the one on your chest.

Why It's Effective: Diaphragmatic breathing engages the diaphragm and has been shown to enhance vagal tone by promoting relaxation and lowering heart rate.(see image)

2. 4-7-8 Breathing Technique

Inhale quietly through the nose for 4 seconds, hold the breath for 7 seconds, and exhale completely through the mouth for 8 seconds.

Why It's Effective: This method is thought to combine elements of mindfulness and physiological relaxation, and it may stimulate the vagus nerve through its prolonged exhalation and breath retention phases.

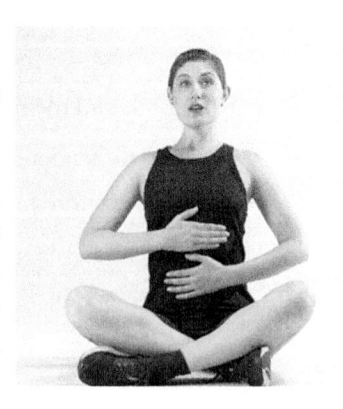

3. Box Breathing (Square Breathing)

Inhale for 4 seconds, hold the breath for 4 seconds, exhale for 4 seconds, and then hold the breath again for 4 seconds.

Why It's Effective: The balanced, rhythmic nature of box breathing helps to regulate the autonomic nervous system and may improve vagal tone by creating a balance between the parasympathetic and sympathetic nervous systems.

4. Alternate Nostril Breathing (Nadi Shodhana)

Close the right nostril with the right thumb and inhale through the left nostril. Close the left nostril with the right ring finger, open the right nostril, and exhale. Inhale through the right nostril, close it, open the left nostril, and exhale.

Why It's Effective: This technique is said to balance the two hemispheres of the brain and regulate the autonomic nervous system, which includes the vagus nerve. It can create a sense of calm and relaxation, thus potentially improving vagal tone.

5. Buteyko Breathing Method

Sit comfortably and take a small, silent breath in and out through your nose. Following the breath, hold your nose to prevent more air from entering. Hold your breath for as long as comfortable. Resume breathing.

Why It's Effective: While primarily used for asthma and other respiratory issues, Buteyko breathing is thought to regulate the balance between oxygen and carbon dioxide, which can stimulate the vagus nerve and contribute to a lowered heart rate and relaxation.

6. The Wim Hof Method:

The Wim Hof Method is a breathing and cold exposure technique developed by Wim Hof, a Dutch extreme athlete. Hof has set multiple world records for enduring extreme cold and holds the belief that his method can enable people to control aspects of their physiology that are typically considered involuntary. The technique has gained international attention and has been subjected to scientific research for its potential benefits on mental and physical health, including improved immune response, stress reduction, increased energy, and even pain relief.

Components of the Wim Hof Method

The Wim Hof Method is mainly built on three pillars:

- Breathing Exercises: A specific form of hyperventilation and breath retention.
- Cold Exposure: Cold showers or immersion in ice-cold water.
- Meditation/Mindfulness: A focus on mental quietude and body awareness.

How to Do It

Breathing Exercise

- Preparation: Sit or lie down in a comfortable place where you won't be disturbed. Make sure you're on an empty stomach or have eaten lightly.

- Phase 1 - Controlled Hyperventilation: Inhale deeply through the nose or mouth, filling the lungs completely, and then exhale without forcing, letting the breath go naturally. Repeat this 30 to 40 times. You might feel light-headed, tingly, or euphoric; these sensations are generally considered normal.
- Phase 2 - Breath Retention: After the final exhale, hold your breath for as long as you comfortably can. The aim is not to push yourself to the limit but to hold the breath until you feel the urge to breathe again.
- Phase 3 - Recovery Breath: Inhale deeply and hold for about 15-20 seconds before exhaling. This marks the end of one round.
- Perform about 3-4 rounds of this breathing cycle.

Cold Exposure

- Starting Small: If you're new to cold exposure, start with a regular shower and then turn the water to cold for the last 30 seconds.
- Gradual Increase: Gradually increase the time you spend under cold water. Advanced practitioners can work their way up to ice baths.

Meditation/Mindfulness

- Focus: During both the breathing exercises and cold exposure, focus your mind on the sensations in your body and try to be aware of every inhale, exhale, and the feeling of the cold against your skin.

Why It's Effective Physiological Benefits
- Increased Oxygen Levels: The hyperventilation phase increases oxygen levels in the blood, which may result in enhanced cellular function and energy.
- Improved Immune Response: Some research suggests the method can modulate the immune system, making it more effective in fighting off pathogens.
- Stress Reduction: The method is thought to influence the autonomic nervous system, helping individuals better manage stress.

Mental Benefits

- Increased Mindfulness: The focus on breath and body sensation enhances mindfulness, which has its own set of well-documented benefits like improved mental clarity and stress reduction.

Vagal Tone
- The combination of controlled breathing and cold exposure is thought to stimulate the vagus nerve, improving vagal tone, which is associated with a range of health benefits including better stress response, reduced inflammation, and improved emotional well-being.

Precautions
- The Wim Hof Method is generally considered safe for healthy individuals but should be practiced with caution. People with cardiovascular issues, high blood pressure, or other serious health conditions should consult a healthcare provider before attempting the technique.

Note: The method requires proper training, preferably under the guidance of certified instructors, especially for those new to the practice. Always prioritize safety and listen to your body's signals.

7. Ocean's Breath (Ujjayi Breathing)

How to Do It: Sit in a comfortable position, keeping your back straight. Inhale deeply through your nose.

As you exhale, slightly constrict the back of your throat. This should create a soft, ocean-like sound as the air passes through. Imagine you are trying to fog up a mirror or sound like Darth Vader. This method activates the vocal cords which are innervated by the vagus nerve.

8. Bhramari Breathing (Bee Breath)

How to Do It: Sit comfortably with your back straight.

Close your eyes and take a deep breath in. As you exhale, use your thumbs to close off your ears.

Keeping your ears closed, make a humming sound like a bee as you exhale. The humming sound and ear canal pressure are believed to stimulate the vagus nerve, which in turn could help improve its tone.

9. Combined Ujjayi-Bhramari Breathing Exercise

Duration: Around 10 minutes for beginners; can be extended as you get more comfortable.

How to Do It: Sit in a comfortable meditative posture, keeping your spine straight and shoulders relaxed. Take a few normal breaths to center yourself.

1. Initial Ujjayi Breath: Inhale deeply through your nose, slightly constricting the back of your throat to produce the ocean-like sound.
2. Transition: Close your ears with your thumbs while holding your breath momentarily.
3. Bhramari Exhale: Keeping your ears closed, make the humming sound like a bee as you exhale.
4. Return: Release your thumbs and return to normal breathing for a few moments.
5. Cycle: Repeat the combined Ujjayi-Bhramari breaths for about 10 rounds or more as you get comfortable.

Augment Vagal Tone from Home: Meditation

The Integrated Vagal-Tone Enhancing Meditation (IVTEM)

IVTEM is a groundbreaking form of meditation and mindfulness practice that synergistically combines elements from ten different established methods, aiming to holistically improve vagal tone. This comprehensive approach also incorporates the use of an eye pillow for ocular stimulation, offering a multi-sensory experience designed to optimize vagus nerve activation.

Components:
1. Loving-Kindness Meditation
2. Progressive Muscle Relaxation

3. Mindful Breathing
4. Body Scan Meditation
5. Ocular Stimulation via Eye Pillow

Duration: 30 minutes

Equipment Needed:
- A comfortable sitting or lying position
- An eye pillow (preferably filled with flaxseed or lavender for added relaxation benefits)

Step-by-Step Guide:
1. Preparation (5 minutes): Sit or lie in a comfortable position and place your eye pillow beside you.
2. Mindful Breathing (5 minutes): Begin by focusing solely on your breath. Observe each inhale and exhale without judgment.
3. Progressive Muscle Relaxation (5 minutes): Progressively tense and relax muscle groups, starting from the toes and moving up toward the head.
4. Body Scan (5 minutes): Perform a mindful body scan, starting from the feet and moving upwards, paying close attention to bodily sensations.
5. Ocular Stimulation (5 minutes): Lie down and place the eye pillow gently over your eyes. The slight pressure and darkness will indirectly stimulate the vagus nerve, contributing to overall vagal tone enhancement.
6. Closing and Integration (5 minutes): Slowly remove the eye pillow and come back to your normal state, reflecting on the experience and setting a positive intention for the rest of the day.

Why It's Effective:

Holistic Approach: By integrating different techniques that individually contribute to improving vagal tone, the practice aims for a holistic enhancement of both mind and body wellness.

Ocular Stimulation: The eye pillow's gentle pressure stimulates the vagus nerve's ophthalmic branch, providing a unique route to enhanced vagal tone.

Multi-Sensory: The method engages multiple senses and psychological states, increasing the potential for effective vagus nerve stimulation.

Always consult with a healthcare provider before starting any new wellness practice, especially if you have pre-existing medical conditions. IVTEM is intended to be an innovative method, and its efficacy would need to be verified through scientific study.

Augment Vagal Tone from Home: Other Options

Interpersonal Interaction

Positive social interactions can serve as potent vagal stimuli, corroborating the significance of social connectivity in health.

Gargling

This simple oral intervention, often overlooked, has the potential to modulate the vagus nerve.

Neck Massage

Gentle carotid sinus massage has been indicated in vagal stimulation, though people should exercise caution given potential contraindications.

Mammalian Dive Reflex

The mammalian dive reflex is a primitive reflex found in all mammals, particularly noticeable in marine animals like seals. In humans, when our face is exposed to cold water, our body automatically initiates a series of cardioprotective responses to conserve oxygen and prioritize the brain and heart. This reflex helps to enhance vagal tone.

Mammalian Dive Reflex Exercise for Increasing Vagal Tone:

Procedure:
1. Begin by filling a large bowl or basin with cold water. The water should be as cold as comfortably possible. Adding ice can make it even colder, but make sure it's not too cold to the point of causing pain or discomfort.
2. Sit comfortably in a chair in front of the bowl.
3. Take a few deep breaths to calm yourself.
4. Hold your breath and then immerse your face into the cold water, especially ensuring the areas underneath the eyes and the cheek region are submerged (these areas are dense in trigeminal nerve endings, which are believed to stimulate the reflex).
5. Hold for as long as comfortably possible, then come up and breathe. Start with short durations and gradually increase as you become accustomed to the sensation.
6. Repeat this a few times, always ensuring you come up for air when needed.

Precautions:
- If you have any cardiovascular issues or other significant health conditions, consult a physician before attempting this exercise.
- Do not force yourself to hold your breath to the point of discomfort or pain.
- Make sure you are seated comfortably to prevent any dizziness or loss of balance.
- Never do this exercise in a situation where you could be at risk of drowning, like in a pool or bathtub.
- Avoid performing this exercise after eating a large meal.

How this helps:
- The cold water on the face stimulates the trigeminal nerve which has a connection to the vagus nerve.

- The breath-holding mimics a dive, conserving oxygen.

- The body's response to cold water on the face and breath-holding is to slow down the heart rate and redirect blood to vital organs. This reflex action is influenced by the vagus nerve and thus, repeated practice can increase its tone.

Examples of its effects:

- Reduced heart rate.

- Enhanced parasympathetic dominance, leading to feelings of calm and relaxation post-practice.

- Some people have even reported improved digestion and sleep after incorporating this regularly.

The mammalian dive reflex is one of the various ways to stimulate the vagus nerve and increase its tone. It's simple, cost-effective, and can be done at home. However, always be cautious and mindful when practicing, listening to your body's signals.

Augment Vagal Tone from Home: Singing and Chanting

Singing and chanting can be powerful tools for stimulating the vagus nerve due to their influence on the muscles of the throat and diaphragm. The vagus nerve interfaces with the muscles of the throat, making these vocal activities particularly relevant.

Singing for Increasing Vagal Tone:

Procedure:
1. Begin with simple, warm-up vocal exercises, progressing from low to high pitches.
2. Sing a song, ideally one that requires varied pitches and sustained notes. Songs that require deep breathing and holding notes can be more effective for stimulating the vagus nerve.

3. Focus on diaphragmatic breathing (belly breathing). This engages the diaphragm and ensures better voice control and lung capacity, while also promoting parasympathetic (rest and digest) dominance.

Singing Warm-Up Exercise:

1. Lip Trills: Lip trills help to warm up the voice gently and efficiently. They can be practiced across various scales and are excellent for bridging vocal registers.

How to do it:
- Start by blowing air through closed lips, making them vibrate or "trill".
- Begin at a comfortable low note and slide up and down a five-note scale, while maintaining the lip trill.
- You can use a piano or keyboard as a guide.
- E.g., if you're starting on middle C, you would slide up C-D-E-F-G and back down G-F-E-D-C.
- Gradually extend the range by moving the starting note up or down the keyboard.
- Make sure to keep the breath steady, the throat relaxed, and let the lips buzz freely.

2. Sirens: This exercise allows you to use your full range, from your lowest to your highest note, in a smooth and relaxed manner.

How to do it:
- Start at the lowest comfortable note of your range and slide all the way up to the highest note and then back down.
- It should sound like a siren. The key is to maintain a relaxed and steady breath throughout.

Here are some songs and styles that could be effective when sung:

Traditional Chants: Many traditional chants, whether Gregorian, Tibetan,

or Indian, involve sustained notes that require deep breathing. For instance:
- Gregorian Chants: "Salve Regina" or "Ave Maria"
- Indian Chants: "Om Namah Shivaya" or "Gayatri Mantra"

Hymns & Spiritual: Many hymns or spiritual songs are designed for communal singing and have long phrases suitable for deep breathing.
- "Amazing Grace"
- "Ave Maria" (Schubert version)
- "Hallelujah" by Leonard Cohen

Classical Arias: Classical vocal pieces are designed for powerful vocal delivery and controlled breathing.
- "O Mio Babbino Caro" from Gianni Schicchi by Puccini
- "Nessun Dorma" from Turandot by Puccini

Popular Songs with Long Phrases:
- "The Sound of Silence" by Simon & Garfunkel
- "Bridge Over Troubled Water" by Simon & Garfunkel
- "Unchained Melody" by The Righteous Brothers

Songs Specifically for Vocal Exercises:
- There are countless vocal warm-up tracks and albums dedicated to building vocal strength, resonance, and breath control. While these aren't traditional "songs", they are specifically designed for vocal health.

Remember, the key is to select songs that allow for deep, controlled breathing and that resonate personally with you. Whether it's the lyrics, melody, or rhythm, personal connection to the song can enhance the potential benefits.

Benefits and Explanation:
- The act of producing musical vocal sounds involves the controlled

exhale of breath, activating the diaphragm and the muscles of the larynx and pharynx.

- Diaphragmatic breathing during singing promotes relaxation and increases oxygenation in the blood.
- The vibrations in the throat during singing provide physical stimulation to the vagus nerve.

Chanting for Increasing Vagal Tone:

Procedure:
1. Begin with a comfortable seated posture.
2. Take a few deep breaths to center yourself.
3. Start chanting a mantra, phrase, or simple extended sounds like "Om." The emphasis should be on elongation and vibration of the sound, particularly in the chest and throat region.
4. Maintain diaphragmatic breathing throughout.

Benefits and Explanation:
- Chanting creates resonant vibrations in the throat, which can stimulate the vagus nerve.
- Some chants or mantras have specific tonal frequencies that may resonate with the body's natural frequencies, potentially amplifying the beneficial effects.
- The rhythmic breathing and focused attention during chanting can enhance relaxation and mindfulness, further promoting vagal activity.

Specifics to consider:
- The sound "Om," often used in yogic traditions, is chanted in three parts: "A-U-M." The "A" begins in the back of the throat and is guttural, the "U" moves through the center of the mouth, and the "M" closes the lips, allowing vibrations to resonate in the skull.
- Some believe that the vibrations from "Om" chanting stimulate the vagus nerve, particularly when the sound is produced loudly and

clearly, and the vibrations are felt in the chest and throat.

Precautions:
- Ensure you are in a comfortable environment where you can sing or chant without feeling self-conscious.
- Stay hydrated, as singing and chanting can be drying for the throat.
- As with all breathing-related exercises, be mindful and avoid hyperventilation or breath-holding that leads to discomfort.

Both singing and chanting can be considered natural vagal nerve stimulators. Their effects are multi-dimensional, combining emotional, psychological, and physiological responses, all of which can contribute to increased well-being and enhanced vagal tone.

References

1. Buijze, G.A., Sierevelt, I.N., van der Heijden, B.C., Dijkgraaf, M.G. and Frings-Dresen, M.H., 2016. The Effect of Cold Showering on Health and Work: A Randomized Controlled Trial. PLoS One, 11(9), e0161749. doi:10.1371/journal.pone.0161749. Erratum in: PLoS One, 2018 Aug 2;13(8):e0201978. PMID: 27631616; PMCID: PMC5025014.

2. Billman, G.E., 2011. Heart rate variability - a historical perspective. Front Physiol, 2:86. doi:10.3389/fphys.2011.00086. PMID: 22144961; PMCID: PMC3225923.

3. Cryan, J.F. and Dinan, T.G., 2012. Mind-altering microorganisms: the impact of the gut microbiota on brain and behaviour. Nat Rev Neurosci, 13(10), pp.701-12. doi:10.1038/nrn3346. PMID: 22968153.

4. Kok, B.E., Coffey, K.A., Cohn, M.A., Catalino, L.I., Vacharkulksemsuk, T., Algoe, S.B., Brantley, M. and Fredrickson, B.L., 2013. How positive emotions build physical health: perceived positive social connections account for the upward spiral between positive emotions and vagal tone. Psychol Sci, 24(7), pp.1123-32. doi:10.1177/0956797612470827. Erratum in: Psychol Sci, 2016 Jun;27(6):931. PMID: 23649562.

5. Kreutz, G., Bongard, S., Rohrmann, S., Hodapp, V. and Grebe, D., 2004. Effects of choir singing or listening on secretory immunoglobulin A, cortisol, and emotional state. J Behav Med, 27(6), pp.623-35. doi:10.1007/s10865-004-0006-9. PMID: 15669447.

6. Krygier, J.R., Heathers, J.A., Shahrestani, S., Abbott, M., Gross, J.J. and Kemp, A.H., 2013. Mindfulness meditation, well-being, and heart rate variability: a preliminary investigation into the impact of intensive Vipassana meditation. Int J Psychophysiol, 89(3), pp.305-13. doi:10.1016/j.ijpsycho.2013.06.017. PMID: 23797150.

7. Lehrer, P.M. and Gevirtz, R., 2014. Heart rate variability biofeedback: how and why does it work? Front Psychol, 5:756. doi:10.3389/fpsyg.2014.00756. PMID: 25101026; PMCID: PMC4104929.

8. Panneton, W.M. and Gan, Q., 2020. The Mammalian Diving Response: Inroads to Its Neural Control. Front Neurosci, 14:524. doi:10.3389/fnins.2020.00524. PMID: 32581683; PMCID: PMC7290049.

9. Pasquier, M., Clair, M., Pruvot, E., Hugli, O. and Carron, P.N., 2017. Carotid Sinus Massage. The New England journal of medicine, 377(15).

10. Sloan, R.P., Shapiro, P.A., DeMeersman, R.E., Bagiella, E., Brondolo, E.N., McKinley, P.S., Slavov, I., Fang, Y. and Myers, M.M., 2009. The effect of aerobic training and cardiac autonomic regulation in young adults. Am J Public Health, 99(5), pp.921-8. doi:10.2105/AJPH.2007.133165. PMID: 19299682; PMCID: PMC2667843.

Chapter 28
Detoxification

The vagus nerve, also known as the tenth cranial nerve, plays a crucial role in the body's parasympathetic nervous system. Originating in the brain and extending to the abdomen, the vagus nerve interacts with various organs and regulates involuntary processes like heart rate and digestion. This article explores its multifaceted involvement in toxin elimination, particularly focusing on its roles in the gastrointestinal tract (GIT), liver, kidneys, and brain.

Within the GIT, which often serves as the first line of defense against ingested toxins, the vagus nerve performs several critical functions. For instance, it triggers nausea and vomiting through the emetic reflex when toxic substances are detected, thereby preventing their absorption into the bloodstream. It achieves this by stimulating the area postrema, a part of the brain responsible for emesis. The nerve also facilitates rapid toxin elimination by altering intestinal motility and secretion, which can lead to diarrhea. This heightened parasympathetic signaling expedites the passage of stool and aids in faster toxin removal.

Additionally, the vagus nerve is key in transmitting information between the GIT and the brain, helping the body identify and respond to potential threats. It does this through chemoreceptors and mechanoreceptors along the GIT, which can detect harmful substances and signal the brain to initiate appropriate responses such as vomiting or altered gut motility. The vagus nerve also significantly influences the gut microbiome. Recent research suggests that what appears to be a shift towards a more "pathogenic" microbiome following toxin ingestion may be a protective, intentional physiological response orchestrated by vagal signaling. Such bacterial populations are often better equipped with metabolic pathways capable of neutralizing or eliminating harmful substances, thus enhancing the body's capability for toxin elimination. This nuanced role of the vagus nerve reveals its essential contributions to homeostasis and protective mechanisms in the human body.

Liver Detoxification

The liver serves as the body's primary detoxification organ, filtering the blood to remove a myriad of harmful substances such as toxins, drugs, and metabolic waste. The vagus nerve plays a pivotal role in enhancing the liver's detoxification processes through its parasympathetic fibers, which help regulate liver metabolism. Specifically, the liver engages in two main phases of detoxification: Phase I transforms toxins into less harmful substances via oxidation, reduction, and hydrolysis, while Phase II focuses on conjugation, where these transformed substances are bound with other molecules for easier excretion. The vagus nerve is believed to modulate these metabolic processes, thereby enhancing the liver's efficacy in toxin elimination.

Beyond its role in detoxification, the vagus nerve also impacts the liver's circulatory regulation. It has the ability to influence the hepatic portal system, a complex vascular network responsible for filtering blood through the liver. By modulating vessel dilation and blood flow, the vagus nerve facilitates more efficient detoxification. Additionally, vagal stimulation often leads to gallbladder contraction and the subsequent secretion of bile, which is particularly vital when fats are consumed. The bile not only aids in digestion but also helps to eliminate waste products and toxins from the body. In this way, the vagus nerve serves to coordinate the activities of the liver and gallbladder, such as synchronizing increased bile production in the liver with the gall bladder's emptying of its stores to make room for fresh bile laden with new toxins and waste products.

Vagal Modulation in Detoxification

The vagus nerve acts like a regulatory hub that synchronizes liver and gallbladder activities in real-time.

Adaptive Responses: Upon ingestion or detection of toxins, the vagus nerve can activate adaptive responses in both the liver and gallbladder. For instance, it may stimulate the liver to ramp up Phase I and Phase II detoxification processes and signal the gallbladder to release stored bile, thereby aiding in the rapid elimination of harmful substances.

Feedback Mechanisms: The vagus nerve provides a feedback loop between the liver, gallbladder, and central nervous system. This allows the body to adapt its detoxification efforts based on the current physiological state and the nature of the toxins present.

Renal Filtration and the Vagus Nerve

The kidneys serve as another vital organ system in the body's detoxification arsenal. These bean-shaped organs filter the blood to remove waste products, excess nutrients, electrolytes, excreting them in the form of urine. The vagus nerve, a key player in the autonomic nervous system, has a nuanced relationship with the kidneys that contributes to the body's overall detoxification efforts.

Glomerular Filtration Rate (GFR): The kidneys adjust the rate at which blood is filtered based on physiological needs. While the vagus nerve's direct role in regulating GFR is not as prominent as other regulatory pathways, it does have an indirect influence. By affecting the systemic inflammatory response and neuroendocrine signaling, the vagus nerve can indirectly influence kidney function and, thus, the filtration process.

Vagal Anti-Inflammatory Pathway: The vagus nerve is implicated in controlling systemic inflammation through what's known as the "cholinergic anti-inflammatory pathway." In the context of kidney function, reducing inflammation can help maintain healthy kidney tissues, ensuring optimal filtration and detoxification.

Urine Production and Excretion: The kidneys produce urine as a means to eliminate waste and regulate body fluids. Urine is also a primary route for the body to excrete certain toxins.

Diuresis: The vagus nerve can impact the secretion of hormones like vasopressin, which in turn influence urine production. While most of the hormonal regulation of diuresis is governed by other neural pathways and endocrine organs, the vagus nerve's overall effect on systemic physiology can indirectly affect urine output and, consequently, toxin elimination.

Neuroendocrine Regulation: The vagus nerve contributes to a complex neuroendocrine network that involves multiple organs and systems. Through this network, the vagus nerve can impact renal function indirectly, affecting the kidneys' ability to excrete toxins efficiently.

Detoxification of the Brain Modulated by Vagal Inputs

The brain is a critical organ with very specialized functions, and as such, it has developed multiple mechanisms to protect itself from potentially harmful substances. Some of the key systems and mechanisms that help the brain block toxins and detoxify are:

Blood-Brain Barrier (BBB):

One of the most important defense mechanisms is the blood-brain barrier, a semipermeable membrane that separates the blood from the cerebrospinal fluid and brain extracellular fluid. The BBB is highly selective, allowing only specific molecules like glucose and essential amino acids to pass through while blocking most large molecules and potentially harmful substances, such as bacteria and toxins.

The vagus nerve plays a protective role in attenuating the permeability of the blood-brain barrier (BBB), a critical structure that prevents harmful substances from entering the brain. Possibly, through the "cholinergic anti-inflammatory pathway," thus regulating the release of pro-inflammatory cytokines that otherwise may compromise the integrity of the BBB. Additionally, the vagus nerve modulates the behavior of astrocytes that line the BBB. By modulating inflammation and influencing the release of protective neurotransmitters, the vagus nerve helps to maintain the tight junctions that constitute the BBB, thus serving as an additional layer of defense against the infiltration of toxins into the central nervous system.

Glial Cells:

Astrocytes are a type of glial cell that helps form the blood-brain barrier. They also play a role in detoxifying the brain environment by taking up excess neurotransmitters, ions, and other substances that could be harmful if they accumulate. Astrocytes are influenced by vagal signaling to regulate tight junctions between endothelial cells, enhancing the BBB's selective permeability. This helps in keeping toxins and harmful substances at bay. Furthermore, astrocytes respond to vagal stimulation by modulating the release of neurotrophic factors and anti-inflammatory cytokines, which can have a restorative and protective effect on the neural tissue.

Microglia, another type of glial cell, serve as the "clean-up crew," scavenging dead cells and other debris. Microglia are sensitive to vagal signaling. Vagal activation can dampen the pro-inflammatory response of activated microglia, thereby reducing neuroinflammation and its associated damage. This is part of the broader "cholinergic anti-inflammatory pathway," in which vagal signaling inhibits the release of pro-inflammatory cytokines, thereby conferring a neuroprotective effect. In this manner, the vagus nerve engages both astrocytes and microglia to maintain the BBB and protect the brain from potential damage by toxins and other harmful substances.

Enzymatic Detoxification:

Various enzymes in the brain contribute to detoxification. For example, enzymes like cytochrome P450 in astrocytes metabolize foreign substances and make them easier to eliminate. This enzyme is modulated by the vagus nerve due to its influence over astrocytic behavior.

Antioxidant Systems:

The brain is highly susceptible to oxidative stress due to its high oxygen consumption. To counter this, it has a robust antioxidant system, including molecules like glutathione and enzymes like superoxide dismutase and catalase, which neutralize reactive oxygen species.

The vagus nerve plays a significant role in the body's oxidative stress response, which includes the production of vital antioxidant enzymes like glutathione, superoxide dismutase (SOD), and catalase within the brain. While direct evidence of the vagus nerve specifically modulating these antioxidants is limited, it is well-established that vagal activation influences these enzymes in other organs.

Efflux Transporters:

Certain cellular transporters actively pump out foreign substances from the brain back into the bloodstream, contributing to detoxification. Examples include the P-glycoprotein and multidrug resistance proteins. These proteins can be upregulated in the brain via the vagus nerve according to some research.

Immune Surveillance:

While the brain was once thought to be an "immune-privileged" site, we now know that immune cells like T-cells and dendritic cells do surveil the brain and can mount responses against pathogens and other harmful agents, albeit in a highly regulated manner.

The vagus nerve has been shown to modulate various aspects of immune function, including the activity of T-cells in the brain. This interaction forms part of the neuro-immune axis, where the nervous and immune systems communicate to maintain homeostasis and respond to injury or toxicity. It can transmit signals that affect T-cell migration, activation, and cytokine production, essentially 'instructing' the immune cells on how to respond to various challenges, including those within the brain.

Cerebrospinal Fluid (CSF) Circulation:

The CSF helps in the removal of metabolic waste products and plays a role in immune surveillance. Newer research also suggests that a "glymphatic system" may help in removing waste substances from the brain, particularly during sleep.

Studies have shown that stimulating the vagus nerve enhances the flow of cerebrospinal fluid (CSF) into the brain, which in turn improves the exchange between CSF and the interstitial fluid (ISF). This increased fluid exchange is crucial for more efficient removal of waste products from the brain, thereby aiding in overall brain detoxification and homeostasis.

Protecting the brain from toxins is a complex, multi-layered process involving a range of cellular, biochemical, and physiological mechanisms. Failure in these systems can contribute to various neurological diseases and conditions.

The vagus nerve is integral to toxin elimination. Through its roles in triggering gastrointestinal, liver, kidney, lung and brain responses it is vital in this process. Understanding these roles can aid in medical interventions aimed at enhancing the body's natural defenses against toxins.

References

1. Xie, Z., Zhang, X., Zhao, M., Huo, L., Huang, M., Li, D., Zhang, S., Cheng, X., Gu, H., Zhang, C., Zhan, C., Wang, F., Shang, C., Cao, P., 2022. The gut-to-brain axis for toxin-induced defensive responses. Cell, 185(23), pp.4298-4316.e21. doi:10.1016/j.cell.2022.10.001. PMID: 36323317.

2. McDougal, D.H., Hermann, G.E., Rogers, R.C., 2011. Vagal afferent stimulation activates astrocytes in the nucleus of the solitary tract via AMPA receptors: evidence of an atypical neural-glial interaction in the brainstem. J Neurosci, 31(39), pp.14037-45. doi:10.1523/JNEUROSCI.2855-11.2011. PMID: 21957265; PMCID: PMC3445261.

3. Romanovsky, A.A., Simons, C.T., Kulchitsky, V.A., Sugimoto, N., Székely, M., 1998. Vagus nerve in fever. Recent developments. Ann N Y Acad Sci, 856, pp.298-299. doi:10.1111/j.1749-6632.1998.tb08343.x. PMID: 9917895.

4. Hansen, M.K., O'Connor, K.A., Goehler, L.E., Watkins, L.R., Maier, S.F., 2001. The contribution of the vagus nerve in interleukin-1beta-induced fever is dependent on dose. Am J Physiol Regul Integr Comp Physiol, 280(4), pp.R929-34. doi:10.1152/ajpregu.2001.280.4.R929. PMID: 11247812.

5. Tu, P., Chi, L., Bodnar, W., Zhang, Z., Gao, B., Bian, X., Stewart, J., Fry, R., Lu, K., 2020. Gut Microbiome Toxicity: Connecting the Environment and Gut Microbiome-Associated Diseases. Toxics, 8(1), 19. doi:10.3390/toxics8010019. PMID: 32178396; PMCID: PMC7151736.

6. Xia, H., Liu, Z., Liang, W., Zeng, X., Yang, Y., Chen, P., Zhong, Z., Ye, Q., 2020. Vagus Nerve Stimulation Alleviates Hepatic Ischemia and Reperfusion Injury by Regulating Glutathione Production and Transformation. Oxid Med Cell Longev, 2020, 1079129. doi:10.1155/2020/1079129. PMID: 32064020; PMCID: PMC6996675.

7. Yang, Y., Yang, L.Y., Orban, L., Cuylear, D., Thompson, J., Simon, B., Yang, Y., 2018. Non-invasive vagus nerve stimulation reduces blood-brain

barrier disruption in a rat model of ischemic stroke. Brain Stimul, 11(4), pp.689-698. doi:10.1016/j.brs.2018.01.034. PMID: 29496430; PMCID: PMC6019567.

8. Kaya, M., Orhan, N., Karabacak, E., Bahceci, M.B., Arican, N., Ahishali, B., Kemikler, G., Uslu, A., Cevik, A., Yilmaz, C.U., Kucuk, M., Gürses, C., 2013. Vagus nerve stimulation inhibits seizure activity and protects blood-brain barrier integrity in kindled rats with cortical dysplasia. Life Sci, 92(4-5), pp.289-97. doi:10.1016/j.lfs.2013.01.009. PMID: 23333826.

9. Cheng, K.P., Brodnick, S.K., Blanz, S.L., Zeng, W., Kegel, J., Pisaniello, J.A., Ness, J.P., Ross, E., Nicolai, E.N., Settell, M.L., Trevathan, J.K., Poore, S.O., Suminski, A.J., Williams, J.C., Ludwig, K.A., 2020. Clinically-derived vagus nerve stimulation enhances cerebrospinal fluid penetrance. Brain Stimul, 13(4), pp.1024-1030. doi:10.1016/j.brs.2020.03.012. PMID: 32388045.

Chapter 29
Epilepsy

Vagus nerve stimulation (VNS) has garnered increasing interest in the medical community as an adjunctive therapy for the management of refractory epilepsy. However, despite its clinical application, the exact mechanism by which VNS modulates epileptiform activity remains an intricate puzzle, involving a myriad of neuroanatomical, electrochemical, and neurophysiological components. This complexity is partly due to the multifaceted functions of the vagus nerve itself, a cranial nerve with widespread projections and roles ranging from autonomic control to direct and indirect modulation of cerebral function. This section aims to illuminate the sophisticated mechanism of action of VNS in epilepsy treatment, focusing on four main pillars: the neuroanatomical pathways involved, the electrochemical theories behind its effects on seizure activity, its role in neurotransmitter modulation, and the effects it imposes on brain networks responsible for seizure genesis.

Neuroanatomical Pathway Involved in VNS:

The vagus nerve, the tenth cranial nerve, is an intricate component of the parasympathetic nervous system, with both afferent and efferent fibers. It communicates with several brain regions either directly or via relay stations such as the nucleus of the solitary tract (NTS). Upon electrical stimulation via an implanted VNS device, afferent fibers transmit signals to the NTS, which, in turn, projects to higher brain regions including the thalamus and the limbic system, known substrates for seizure initiation and propagation.

Electrochemical Theories Explaining VNS Impacts on Seizure Activity:

Various electrochemical theories have been posited to elucidate the modulatory effects of VNS on neuronal activity. Among these, one prevailing hypothesis suggests the involvement of ion channels and membrane potential stabilization. Electrical stimulation of the vagus nerve may bring about changes in the conductance of specific ion channels, thereby stabilizing the neuronal membrane and making it less susceptible to erratic depolarization, the hallmark of seizure activity.

Role in Modulating Neurotransmitters:

Beyond ion channel manipulation, VNS is thought to influence the concentration and action of a variety of neurotransmitters, most notably gamma-aminobutyric acid (GABA) and glutamate. The balance between these excitatory and inhibitory neurotransmitters is critical in maintaining a stable neuronal environment. VNS has been demonstrated to augment the release of GABA while attenuating the levels of excitatory amino acids, thereby tipping the balance towards inhibition and potentially averting seizure onset.

Effects on Brain Networks Involved in Seizure Generation:

Finally, the application of VNS appears to have far-reaching effects on brain networks implicated in seizure pathophysiology. Studies involving functional magnetic resonance imaging (fMRI) and electroencephalography (EEG) have provided insights into how VNS may modulate network connectivity, especially within the default mode network and thalamocortical circuits. By affecting long-range connections between these brain regions, VNS could impede the synchronization processes crucial for seizure generation and propagation.

In conclusion, the mechanism of action of VNS in epilepsy is a dynamic interplay of neuroanatomical structures, electrochemical changes, neurotransmitter modulation, and network connectivity adjustments. Understanding these mechanisms not only substantiates the clinical utility of VNS but also offers avenues for refining therapeutic strategies for epilepsy management.

Research on Vagus Nerve Stimulation for Epilepsy

A retrospective study by Boluk et al. (2022) assessed the efficacy and safety of vagus nerve stimulation (VNS) in treating various types of epilepsy from 2005 to 2020. The study involved 41 patients with different forms of epilepsy, including focal, generalized, and combined types like Lennox-Gastaut and Dravet syndrome. Results indicated a significant reduction in seizure frequency across all types of epilepsy at the 12th month after VNS implantation, with a response rate of 68.3%. The number of antiseizure medications also decreased significantly. Adverse events led to the discontinuation of VNS therapy in 4.9% of patients. Despite a low rate of complete seizure freedom, the study concludes that VNS is a safe and effective treatment option for various forms of epilepsy, especially for those not eligible for resective surgery (Boluk et al., 2022).

The study by von Wrede and Surges (2021) reviews the clinical efficacy and safety of transcutaneous vagus nerve stimulation (tVNS) in treating drug-resistant epilepsy. While invasive vagus nerve stimulation (iVNS) is well-established, tVNS offers the advantages of being non-surgical and instantly removable. The paper synthesizes data from five prospective trials and three randomized controlled trials, involving a total of 398 patients. Despite heterogeneity in study designs, results showed promising seizure reduction rates of up to 64%, with responder rates (seizure reduction ≥50%) reaching up to 65%. Seizure freedom was achieved in up to 24% of cases and even up to 31% in a small pediatric group. Adverse side effects were generally mild and included headache, ear pain, and skin alteration. Quality of life metrics also showed significant improvement in two studies, emphasizing the promise of tVNS as an effective and safe treatment option for drug-resistant epilepsy, though the authors call for more standardized and long-term studies to definitively assess its efficacy (von Wrede & Surges, 2021).

In a randomized, double-blind clinical trial by Bauer et al. (2016), the efficacy and safety of transcutaneous vagus nerve stimulation (tVNS) were evaluated in patients with drug-resistant epilepsy. The study compared the effects of 25 Hz tVNS to an active control group with 1 Hz stimulation over a 20-week period. Despite high treatment adherence rates of 88% in the 25 Hz group and 84% in the 1 Hz group, the study could not conclusively prove the superiority of 25 Hz tVNS in reducing seizure frequency. However, a significant reduction in seizure frequency was observed in patients who completed the full treatment period with 25 Hz tVNS (34.2%, p = 0.034). Adverse events, typically mild or moderate, included headache, ear pain, vertigo, and nausea. The authors concluded that while tVNS was well-tolerated and showed promise in reducing seizures, more extensive trials are necessary to confirm its efficacy (Bauer et al., 2016).

References

1. Bauer, S., Baier, H., Baumgartner, C., Bohlmann, K., Fauser, S., Graf, W., Hillenbrand, B., Hirsch, M., Last, C., Lerche, H., Mayer, T., Schulze-Bonhage, A., Steinhoff, B.J., Weber, Y., Hartlep, A., Rosenow, F., Hamer, H.M., 2016. Transcutaneous Vagus Nerve Stimulation (tVNS) for Treatment of Drug-Resistant Epilepsy: A Randomized, Double-Blind Clinical Trial (cMPsE02). Brain Stimul, 9(3), pp.356-363. doi:10.1016/j.brs.2015.11.003. PMID: 27033012.

2. Boluk, C., Ozkara, C., Isler, C., Uzan, M., 2022. Vagus Nerve Stimulation in Intractable Epilepsy. Turk Neurosurg, 32(1), pp.97-102. doi:10.5137/1019-5149.JTN.33775-21.2. PMID: 34664698.

3. von Wrede, R., Surges, R., 2021. Transcutaneous vagus nerve stimulation in the treatment of drug-resistant epilepsy. Auton Neurosci, 235, 102840. doi:10.1016/j.autneu.2021.102840. PMID: 34246121.

Chapter 30
Atrial Fibrillation

Vagus nerve stimulation (VNS) serves as a compelling modality in the therapeutic armamentarium against atrial fibrillation (AF), a prevalent cardiac arrhythmia characterized by erratic atrial electrical activity and hemodynamic instability. The vagus nerve, as an integral component of the cardiac autonomic nervous system, possesses both afferent and efferent fibers that interface directly with the myocardium, providing a physiological conduit for modulating atrial electrophysiology. Through low-level tragus stimulation, a specific form of VNS, it is possible to engender a perturbation in the intrinsic cardiac neural network, thereby mitigating the substrate conducive to AF initiation and perpetuation.

Mechanistically, VNS has been posited to induce anti-arrhythmic effects via multifaceted pathways. Firstly, it elicits alterations in autonomic tone, favoring parasympathetic predominance that mediates atrial refractory period prolongation. This refractory period modulation engenders a decrement in the wavelength of the reentrant circuits, culminating in arrhythmia termination. Secondly, VNS has demonstrated a capability to modulate ion channel expression and function, particularly affecting the balance between inward and outward currents during the cardiac action potential, thereby stabilizing atrial electrical activity.

Research on VNS for Atrial Fibrillation:

In a sham-controlled, double-blind, randomized clinical trial conducted by Stavrakis et al. (2020), the chronic effects of low-level tragus stimulation (LLTS) on patients with paroxysmal atrial fibrillation (AF) were examined. The study found that after 6 months, the median AF burden was 85% lower in the group receiving active LLTS compared to the sham control group. Additionally, levels of the inflammatory cytokine tumor necrosis factor-alpha were significantly reduced by 23% in the active group. Frequency domain indices of heart rate variability also showed significant changes favoring the active treatment. The study concluded that chronic, intermittent LLTS could be an effective and safe treatment for reducing AF burden in selected patients (Stavrakis et al., 2020; JACC Clin Electrophysiol, 6(3), 282-291).

In a study conducted by Kulkarni et al. (2021), the authors investigated the role of low-level tragus stimulation (LLTS) in managing atrial fibrillation (AF) burden and examined the potential of P-wave alternans (PWA) as a guiding marker for treatment. PWA refers to variations in the P-wave amplitude or morphology on an electrocardiogram and is thought to arise from the same substrate responsible for AF, making it a potentially useful indicator for treatment efficacy. The study discovered that acute LLTS initially led to an increase in PWA burden. However, chronic, intermittent LLTS over 6 months significantly reduced both PWA and AF burden, as compared to a sham control group. These findings indicate that PWA could serve as a valuable marker for optimizing LLTS therapy in the treatment of paroxysmal AF (Kulkarni et al., 2021)

Kharbanda et al. (2022) explored the complex influence of the cardiac autonomic nervous system (CANS) on atrial fibrillation (AF), focusing on the dual pro-arrhythmogenic and anti-arrhythmogenic effects of vagus nerve stimulation (VNS). The study underscored the importance of the anatomical site and settings of VNS in shaping its impact on cardiac electrophysiology. It highlighted the potential of low-level VNS (LLVNS), a form of VNS below the bradycardia threshold, as a promising treatment for AF due to its significant anti-arrhythmic effects. The authors concluded that further research is necessary to understand the underlying anti-arrhythmogenic mechanisms and to optimize the settings and sites for LLVNS in treating AF patients (Kharbanda et al., 2022).

References

1. Stavrakis, S., Stoner, J.A., Humphrey, M.B., Morris, L., Filiberti, A., Reynolds, J.C., Elkholey, K., Javed, I., Twidale, N., Riha, P., Varahan, S., Scherlag, B.J., Jackman, W.M., Dasari, T.W. and Po, S.S., 2020. TREAT AF (Transcutaneous Electrical Vagus Nerve Stimulation to Suppress Atrial Fibrillation): A Randomized Clinical Trial. *JACC Clin Electrophysiol*, 6(3), pp.282-291. doi: 10.1016/j.jacep.2019.11.008. Epub 2020 Jan 29. PMID: 32192678; PMCID: PMC7100921.

2. Kharbanda, R.K., van der Does, W.F.B., van Staveren, L.N., Taverne, Y.J.H.J., Bogers, A.J.J.C., de Groot, N.M.S., 2022. Vagus Nerve Stimulation and Atrial Fibrillation: Revealing the Paradox. Neuromodulation, 25(3), pp.356-365. doi:10.1016/j.neurom.2022.01.008. PMID: 35190246.

3. Kulkarni, K., Singh, J.P., Parks, K.A., Katritsis, D.G., Stavrakis, S., Armoundas, A.A., 2021. Low-Level Tragus Stimulation Modulates Atrial Alternans and Fibrillation Burden in Patients With Paroxysmal Atrial Fibrillation. J Am Heart Assoc, 10(12), e020865. doi:10.1161/JAHA.120.020865. PMID: 34075778; PMCID: PMC8477868.

Chapter 31
Migraine

Vagus nerve stimulation (VNS) has emerged as an innovative neuromodulatory approach in the prophylactic and symptomatic treatment of migraine, a debilitating neurovascular disorder characterized by recurrent episodes of severe headache, photophobia, and phonophobia. As part of the complex cholinergic network, the vagus nerve plays a pivotal role in modulating pain perception and inflammatory response, thereby offering a targetable pathway for migraine amelioration. The vagal afferents are intricately involved in the nociceptive pathways and connect to the trigeminocervical complex, which is implicated in migraine pathophysiology.

Mechanistically, VNS acts through the activation of vagal afferents that synapse on the nucleus tractus solitarius (NTS). From the NTS, secondary neurons relay signals to key areas implicated in migraine pathophysiology such as the locus coeruleus and the dorsal raphe nucleus. Activation of these nuclei culminates in the release of neurotransmitters like serotonin and norepinephrine, which have been implicated in modulating pain transmission. Additionally, VNS has demonstrated anti-inflammatory effects by suppressing the production of pro-inflammatory cytokines such as tumor necrosis factor-alpha (TNF-α), interleukin-1β (IL-1β), and interleukin-6 (IL-6) via the cholinergic anti-inflammatory pathway, thereby attenuating the neurogenic inflammation commonly observed in migraine.

Furthermore, there is compelling evidence to suggest that VNS may modulate cortical spreading depression (CSD), a phenomenon considered pivotal in the genesis of migraine aura and possibly the headache phase. Through neuromodulatory effects on cortical excitability, VNS may prevent the initiation or propagation of CSD, thus attenuating one of the central mechanisms of migraine pathogenesis.

Research on VNS for Migraine:

The systematic review and meta-analysis by Song et al. (2023) evaluates the efficacy and safety of non-invasive vagus nerve stimulation (n-VNS) in treating migraines. The study differentiates between non-invasive cervical VNS (n-cVNS) and non-invasive auricular VNS (n-aVNS), finding that while n-cVNS improved the ≥50% responder rate, it did not significantly reduce the number of migraine or headache days. In contrast, n-aVNS significantly reduced both migraine days and headache intensity but had no impact on the number of acute medication days per month. Overall, n-VNS was found to be a safe and promising non-pharmacological treatment for migraines, although its effectiveness varies depending on the type and parameters of the stimulation used (Song et al., 2023).

In a study conducted by Zhang et al. (2021), 70 migraine patients were randomized to undergo either real or sham transcutaneous auricular vagus nerve stimulation (taVNS) treatments for 4 weeks. Results from the 59 patients who completed the study showed that taVNS significantly reduced the number of migraine days, pain intensity, and migraine attack frequency compared to sham treatment. Functional MRI scans further revealed that taVNS altered thalamocortical connectivity, specifically increasing connectivity between motor-related thalamic subregions and the anterior cingulate cortex/medial prefrontal cortex while decreasing connectivity between occipital cortex-related thalamic subregions and the postcentral gyrus/precuneus. These findings suggest that taVNS not only alleviates migraine symptoms but also modulates relevant neural circuits, offering new therapeutic avenues for migraine treatment (Zhang et al., 2021).

In a multicenter, randomized, double-blind study led by Najib et al. (2022), non-invasive vagus nerve stimulation was evaluated for its efficacy in preventing migraines. Of the 336 adults initially enrolled, 113 completed the study and adhered sufficiently to the treatment regimen. Though the study was prematurely terminated due to the COVID-19 pandemic, the data showed a greater reduction in monthly migraine days in the active treatment group compared to the sham group, although the difference was not statistically significant (mean reduction of 3.12 vs. 2.29 days, p=0.2329). However, the responder rate—defined as participants experiencing at least a 50% reduction in monthly migraine days—was significantly higher in the active group (44.87% vs. 26.81%, p=0.0481). The therapy was particularly effective for patients with migraine with aura and showed a well-established safety profile, with no serious device-related adverse events reported (Najib et al., 2022).

References

1. Najib, U., Smith, T., Hindiyeh, N., Saper, J., Nye, B., Ashina, S., McClure, C.K., Marmura, M.J., Chase, S., Liebler, E., Lipton, R.B., 2022. Non-invasive vagus nerve stimulation for prevention of migraine: The multicenter, randomized, double-blind, sham-controlled PREMIUM II trial. Cephalalgia, 42(7), pp.560-569. doi:10.1177/03331024211068813. PMID: 35001643.

2. Song, D., Li, P., Wang, Y., Cao, J., 2023. Noninvasive vagus nerve stimulation for migraine: a systematic review and meta-analysis of randomized controlled trials. Front Neurol, 14, 1190062. doi:10.3389/fneur.2023.1190062. PMID: 37251233; PMCID: PMC10213755.

3. Zhang Y, Huang Y, Li H, Yan Z, Zhang Y, Liu X, Hou X, Chen W, Tu Y, Hodges S, Chen H, Liu B, Kong J. Transcutaneous auricular vagus nerve stimulation (taVNS) for migraine: an fMRI study. Reg Anesth Pain Med. 2021 Feb;46(2):145-150. doi: 10.1136/rapm-2020-102088. Epub 2020 Dec 1. PMID: 33262253.

Chapter 32
Depression

Vagus nerve stimulation (VNS) represents an avant-garde paradigm in the therapeutic modalities for major depressive disorder (MDD), a psychological affliction characterized by pervasive low mood, anhedonia, and cognitive impairments. Afferent and efferent fibers of the vagus nerve interface with a myriad of central nervous system structures implicated in emotional regulation, including but not limited to the amygdala, dorsal raphe, and locus coeruleus. As such, the vagus nerve serves as an anatomical and functional conduit through which neuromodulatory effects can be disseminated to ameliorate depressive symptomatology.

Mechanistically, VNS exerts its antidepressant effects through multifarious pathways. The activation of vagal afferents has been shown to stimulate the nucleus tractus solitarius (NTS), which in turn interfaces with the noradrenergic locus coeruleus and serotonergic dorsal raphe nuclei. The consequent release of neurotransmitters such as serotonin and norepinephrine in brain regions like the prefrontal cortex has been hypothesized to ameliorate depressive symptoms by enhancing mood-regulatory neurotransmission.

Furthermore, VNS may also play a significant role in modulating neural plasticity through the release of neurotrophic factors such as brain-derived neurotrophic factor (BDNF), thereby contributing to the resilience of neural networks against stress-induced remodeling— a hallmark of depressive pathophysiology. Additionally, VNS has been postulated to influence the hypothalamic-pituitary-adrenal (HPA) axis, mitigating the hyperactivity often observed in depression, which, in turn, can normalize aberrant cortisol levels and reduce neuroinflammation.

VNS's anti-inflammatory properties also extend to the suppression of pro-inflammatory cytokines like interleukin-6 (IL-6) and tumor necrosis factor-alpha (TNF-α) via the cholinergic anti-inflammatory pathway. Given that depression has been increasingly recognized as a neuroinflammatory condition, this anti-inflammatory action adds another layer to VNS's therapeutic potential.

Research on VNS for Depression:

The meta-analysis conducted by Zhang et al. (2020) investigated the efficacy and safety of using vagus nerve stimulation (VNS) as an adjunctive treatment for treatment-resistant depression (TRD). Three controlled studies involving a total of 1048 patients were analyzed, with 622 patients in the VNS group and 426 in the control group. The findings suggest that VNS may be an effective and relatively safe option for treating TRD. The study showed that VNS had a significant impact on treating TRD, with a Standardized Mean Difference (SMD) of 1.96 (95% CI: 1.60, 2.40, $P < 0.00001$). This indicates that patients treated with VNS showed a statistically significant improvement in depression symptoms compared to those in the control group (Zhang et al., 2020).

The meta-analysis supports the idea that adjunctive VNS could be an effective and relatively safe treatment for TRD. However, the limited number of high-quality studies included in the meta-analysis and the high heterogeneity regarding discontinuation rates indicate that further randomized controlled trials are needed to confirm these findings (Zhang et al., 2020).

In a prospective 12-week, single-blind trial led by Li et al. (2022), the efficacy of transcutaneous auricular vagus nerve stimulation (taVNS) was compared to citalopram, a standard antidepressant, in treating Major Depressive Disorder (MDD) in 107 patients. Patients were randomized into either an eight-week taVNS regimen with a four-week follow-up or a 12-week regimen of citalopram (40 mg/d). Both treatments led to reduced Hamilton Depression Rating Scale (HAM-D17) scores, but there was no statistically significant difference between the two groups in terms of this primary outcome (p=0.79). However, taVNS demonstrated a significantly higher remission rate at weeks four and six compared to citalopram. Peripheral blood levels of key neurotransmitters like serotonin, dopamine, GABA, and noradrenaline also changed significantly in both groups but with no significant differences between them. The study concluded that taVNS was as effective as citalopram for treating MDD and should be considered a viable therapeutic option, though the possibility of a placebo effect affecting both groups could not be ruled out (Li et al., 2022).

According to the study by Zhang et al. (2023), Transcutaneous electrical cranial-auricular acupoint stimulation (TECAS) was found to be non-inferior to escitalopram in treating mild-to-moderate major depressive disorder, with comparable clinical response rates and fewer adverse events. TECAS also showed particular efficacy in individuals who had experienced psychological trauma, suggesting it could be a safer, more portable, and effective alternative for certain populations (Zhang et al., 2023).

References

1. Li, S., Rong, P., Wang, Y., Jin, G., hou, X., Li, S., Xiao, X., Zhou, W., Wu, Y., Liu, Y., Zhang, Y., Zhao, B., Huang, Y., Cao, J., Chen, H., Hodges, S., Vangel, M., Kong, J., 2022. Comparative Effectiveness of Transcutaneous Auricular Vagus Nerve Stimulation vs Citalopram for Major Depressive Disorder: A Randomized Trial. Neuromodulation, 25(3), pp.450-460. doi:10.1016/j.neurom.2021.10.021. PMID: 35088753.

2. Ma, Y., He, J., Lu, X., Sun, J., Guo, C., Luo, Y., Gao, S., Liu, Y., Zhang, Z., Rong, P. and Fang, J., 2023. Transcutaneous electrical cranial-auricular acupoint stimulation versus escitalopram for modulating the brain activity in mild to moderate major depressive disorder: An fMRI study. Neurosci Lett., 814, p.137414.

3. Rong, P.J., Fang, J.L., Wang, L.P., Meng, H., Liu, J., Ma, Y.G., Ben, H., Li, L., Liu, R.P., huang, Z.X., Zhao, Y.F., Li, X., Zhu, B., Kong, J., 2012. Transcutaneous vagus nerve stimulation for the treatment of depression: a study protocol for a double-blinded randomized clinical trial. BMC Complement Altern Med, 12, 255. doi:10.1186/1472-6882-12-255. PMID: 23241431; PMCID: PMC3537743.

4. Zhang, X., Qing, M.J., Rao, Y.H. and Guo, Y.M., 2020. Adjunctive Vagus Nerve Stimulation for Treatment-Resistant Depression: a Quantitative Analysis. Psychiatr Q., 91(3), pp.669-679.

.

Chapter 33
Postural Orthostatic Tachycardia Syndrome

Postural Orthostatic Tachycardia Syndrome (POTS) is a multifaceted dysautonomic condition that manifests with symptoms like palpitations, dizziness, and fatigue upon transitioning from a supine to an upright position. As complex as its clinical presentation, the underlying etiology of POTS is equally intricate, with growing evidence pointing towards a role of vagus nerve dysfunction.

The diagnosis of POTS is primarily confirmed through specialized tests such as the tilt-table test or a standing test. These tests monitor both heart rate and blood pressure as the patient transitions from a lying-down to a standing position. The widely accepted diagnostic criteria stipulate that a diagnosis of POTS can be considered if there is either a heart rate increase of at least 30 beats per minute within 10 minutes of moving from lying down to standing up, or if there is a sustained heart rate exceeding 120 beats per minute within the same time frame upon standing. Importantly, these symptoms must be persistent for at least six months and should not be attributable to other causative factors like medications or acute dehydration. It's also worth noting that the diagnostic criteria can differ slightly for children and adolescents, accounting for age-related physiological variations. This stringent set of criteria aims to ensure accurate diagnosis and differentiation from other conditions that may exhibit similar symptoms.

While the underlying pathophysiology of POTS remains a subject of ongoing research and debate, increasing evidence suggests a role for immune system dysfunction in the condition. One indicative factor is the female predominance in POTS cases, as the syndrome is more commonly diagnosed in women and often initiates after events like acute viral infections, vaccinations, or trauma—features that are commonly seen in autoimmune diseases. Furthermore, autoimmune markers lend additional support to the theory of immune involvement; approximately one in four POTS patients test positive for anti-nuclear antibodies, and about 20% have a history of autoimmune disorders such as Hashimoto's thyroiditis or rheumatoid arthritis.

Recent studies have also identified various autoantibodies that may be implicated in POTS. These include autoantibodies against cardiovascular G-protein-coupled membrane complexes like adrenergic, muscarinic, and angiotensin II type-1 receptors. Additional autoantibodies against nicotinic acetylcholine receptors in autonomic ganglia and Sjögren autoantibodies have been found. The presence of these autoantibodies, along with the diverse symptomatology seen in POTS patients, suggests a generalized immune system dysfunction, potentially making these individuals more susceptible to autoimmune disorders. This emerging immunological perspective adds another layer to our understanding of this complex syndrome.

Vagus Nerve Dysfunction in POTS:

Vagus nerve dysfunction can be intertwined with the immunological aspects of POTS. The vagus nerve is integral in maintaining autonomic balance, and its dysfunction can lead to a series of symptoms common in POTS, such as tachycardia, gastrointestinal issues, and fatigue. Dysfunction in the vagus nerve could result from or contribute to the immune dysregulation observed in POTS, although this relationship is yet to be conclusively established.

POTS Management

Management of POTS is multi-faceted and often tailored to individual patient needs, incorporating both lifestyle and pharmacological interventions. Lifestyle modifications form the cornerstone of POTS management and commonly include increased fluid and salt intake to help maintain blood volume, as well as physical conditioning to improve autonomic function and reduce symptoms. Pharmacotherapy is another key element, with medications such as beta-blockers, fludrocortisone, and pyridostigmine frequently prescribed to manage heart rate, blood volume, and autonomic imbalances.

Given the emerging evidence for immune dysfunction in POTS, immunotherapy options like intravenous immunoglobulin (IVIG) are sometimes considered, especially in cases with a suspected autoimmune component. Finally, addressing vagus nerve dysfunction has shown promise in alleviating symptoms. Approaches include transcutaneous vagus nerve stimulation, which involves sending mild electrical impulses to the vagus nerve, and cervical stability rehabilitation to alleviate any mechanical compression affecting the nerve. Collectively, these multidisciplinary treatment approaches aim to manage the complex symptomatology of POTS, offering patients a comprehensive strategy for improving their quality of life.

Conclusion:

POTS is a complex condition with a diverse clinical presentation. Its diagnosis is largely clinical, based on well-defined criteria involving orthostatic intolerance and tachycardia. Emerging evidence suggests a significant role of immune dysfunction, possibly of autoimmune origin, in its pathogenesis. Understanding the immunological aspects and the role of vagus nerve dysfunction in POTS can pave the way for targeted therapies and better management of this debilitating condition.

References

1. Deng, J., Li, H., Guo, Y., Zhang, G., Fischer, H., Stavrakis, S. and Yu, X., 2023. Transcutaneous vagus nerve stimulation attenuates autoantibody-mediated cardiovagal dysfunction and inflammation in a rabbit model of postural tachycardia syndrome. J Interv Card Electrophysiol, 66(2), pp.291-300.

2. Fedorowski, A., 2019. Postural orthostatic tachycardia syndrome: clinical presentation, aetiology and management. J Intern Med, 285(4), pp.352-366.

3. Jacob, G., Diedrich, L., Sato, K., Brychta, R.J., Raj, S.R., Robertson, D., Biaggioni, I. and Diedrich, A., 2019. Vagal and Sympathetic Function in Neuropathic Postural Tachycardia Syndrome. Hypertension, 73(5), pp.1087-1096.

4. Sebastian, S.A., Co, E.L., Panthangi, V., Jain, E., Ishak, A., Shah, Y., Vasavada, A. and Padda, I., 2022. Postural Orthostatic Tachycardia Syndrome (POTS): An Update for Clinical Practice. Curr Probl Cardiol, 47(12), p.101384.

Chapter 34
Ehlers-Danlos Syndrome

Ehlers-Danlos Syndrome (EDS) represents a complex group of connective tissue disorders involving multiple systems within the body. The disorders are largely inherited and exhibit a broad range of phenotypic expression. In 2017, the International EDS Consortium revised the classification system, identifying 13 subtypes of EDS, to replace the older Villefranche and Berlin systems. This updated classification not only provides more specific diagnostic criteria but also includes recommendations for genetic and molecular confirmatory tests for each subtype, except for the hypermobile type. This review will delve into each subtype and also discuss Hypermobility Spectrum Disorders (HSD) as a related condition.

EDS Subtypes

Ehlers-Danlos Syndrome (EDS) is classified into various subtypes, each with its own set of major and minor diagnostic criteria. Classical EDS is defined by major criteria such as atrophic scarring, skin hyperextensibility, and generalized joint hypermobility, while minor criteria include elements like epicanthic folds, skin fragility, easy bruising, and a family history of the disorder. Classical-like EDS shares some similarities, featuring skin hyperextensibility and generalized joint hypermobility but lacks atrophic scarring as a major criterion. Its minor criteria range from non-cardiogenic lower extremity edema to mild muscle weakness and axonal polyneuropathy.

Cardiac-valvular EDS distinguishes itself primarily through progressive cardiac-valvular problems, along with skin hyperextensibility, atrophic scarring, and joint hypermobility. Minor criteria for this subtype can include foot deformities and joint dislocations. Vascular EDS is particularly severe and is characterized by major criteria like arterial rupture at a young age and uterine rupture, with minor criteria such as congenital hip dislocation. Hypermobile EDS is unique in that it has no known associated gene mutations and is entirely a clinical diagnosis requiring three strict criteria to be met.

In addition to these, the 2017 classification system also enumerates other lesser-known subtypes of EDS, each with its unique set of diagnostic criteria. These include dermatosparaxis, kyphoscoliotic, brittle cornea syndrome, spondylodysplastic, musculocontractural, myopathic, periodontal, and arthrochalasia types. The detailed diagnostic criteria for each of these are elaborated in the 2017 classification, making EDS a complex and multifaceted disorder requiring nuanced diagnosis.

EDS Diagnosis

The diagnosis of Ehlers-Danlos Syndrome is a comprehensive, multi-step process that involves clinical evaluation, family history assessment, physical examination, and specialized tests including genetic testing where appropriate. Due to the broad range of phenotypic expressions and multiple subtypes, the process requires meticulous care.

Preliminary screening for Ehlers-Danlos Syndrome (EDS) involves a multi-step approach to collect comprehensive information for diagnosis. The process often begins with a thorough patient history and symptom assessment, where clinicians delve into details like skin elasticity, easy bruising, history of joint dislocations, and other symptoms relevant to EDS. This initial assessment lays the groundwork for understanding the patient's condition and guides further diagnostic measures. Equally important is a detailed family history, as EDS can have hereditary patterns. Obtaining a family history is crucial for assessing the pattern of inheritance and identifying other family members who may have undiagnosed EDS, thereby providing invaluable context for the patient's symptoms.

Following these history assessments, a physical examination is usually conducted, honing in on hallmark features of the syndrome. This includes tests for skin elasticity, inspections for scarring, and evaluations of joint mobility, among other criteria. The information collected during this physical examination is then used in conjunction with the patient's history to make an informed diagnostic decision, possibly leading to further specialized tests based on the suspected EDS subtype. These preliminary screening steps are fundamental in ensuring a nuanced and accurate diagnosis of this complex and multifaceted disorder.

Specialized Tests

Brighton Criteria for Joint Hypermobility: The Brighton Criteria commonly referred to as the Brighton Scale, serves as a diagnostic standard for identifying Joint Hypermobility Syndrome (JHS), often considered a variant or closely related to Ehlers-Danlos Syndrome (EDS). Designed to provide diagnostic uniformity, especially in subtle or ambiguous cases, the Brighton Criteria evaluate not only the range of joint movements but also include factors such as skin texture, systemic symptoms, and familial history of hypermobility or related conditions.

The Brighton Criteria include both major and minor criteria. For a diagnosis using the Brighton Criteria, a patient must meet one of the following sets of conditions:

- Fulfill two major criteria
- Fulfill one major criterion and two minor criteria
- Fulfill four minor criteria
- Have two minor criteria plus at least two first-degree relatives (either parents, siblings, or children) meeting one of the first three conditions

Major Criteria:

Brighton Criteria of 4 or Higher: The Brighton Criteria quantifies joint hypermobility on a scale of 0 to 9 and involves several tests of specific joint movements:

- Passive dorsiflexion of the fifth finger beyond 90 degrees
- Passive apposition of the thumb to the flexor aspect of the forearm
- Hyperextension of the elbows beyond 10 degrees
- Hyperextension of the knees beyond 10 degrees
- Ability to place the palms on the floor while bending forward, with knees fully extended
- Arthralgia for Longer Than 3 Months: This involves experiencing joint pain in one or more joints for an extended period.

Minor Criteria:

- Brighton Criteria of 1-3: Or a score of 0-3 for individuals aged 50 or older.
- Arthralgia in up to 3 Joints or Back Pain: Persisting for more than three months.
- Joint Subluxation or Dislocation: Either in more than one joint or the same joint on multiple occasions.
- Soft Tissue Rheumatism: Such as bursitis or tenosynovitis.
- Marfanoid Habitus: Characteristics include a tall, slim physique, arm span to height ratio greater than 1.03, and other specific features.
- Skin Stigmata: Such as abnormal scarring or thin, hyper-elastic skin.
- Eye Signs: Including myopia or drooping eyelids.
- Vascular Complications: Such as varicose veins, hernia, or uterine/rectal prolapse.

Utility and Limitations:

The Brighton Criteria serve as a comprehensive tool to diagnose JHS and conditions that fall under the broader hypermobility spectrum. They are particularly helpful for diagnosing older adults whose joint flexibility may have decreased with age. However, the criteria are not aligned with the latest 2017 EDS classification and don't specifically include genetic markers, which are increasingly important for a comprehensive diagnosis.

Beyond the Brighton Criteria commonly used for diagnosing Ehlers-Danlos Syndrome (EDS), additional diagnostic avenues can further refine the understanding of the condition. Imaging tests like X-rays and MRIs serve as useful supplementary tools for evaluating skeletal abnormalities and joint issues. Although these tests are not definitive for diagnosing EDS, they can provide valuable insights into the extent of structural anomalies, thereby aiding the diagnostic process. In the realm of molecular genetics, specific tests are available for many EDS subtypes. By analyzing blood samples, mutations in genes associated with different subtypes can be identified, adding another layer of diagnostic precision. It's important to note, however, that hypermobile EDS currently lacks a genetic marker, making it solely a clinical diagnosis based on symptoms and physical examination.

Given the symptomatic overlap between EDS and other connective tissue disorders, differential diagnosis becomes a critical component of the evaluation. Conditions like Marfan Syndrome, Loeys-Dietz Syndrome, and Osteogenesis Imperfecta can present with similar features, making it crucial to rule them out for an accurate EDS diagnosis. This multi-faceted approach, incorporating both clinical and specialized tests, ensures a more comprehensive and accurate diagnostic process for this complex condition.

Clinical Criteria for Subtype Identification:

The 2017 classification system has set specific major and minor criteria for each subtype of EDS. A diagnosis of a specific subtype usually involves meeting a certain number of these criteria. For example, the Classical EDS subtype requires the presence of specific major criteria like atrophic scarring and skin hyperextensibility, as well as some minor criteria for a conclusive diagnosis.

Genetics and Aetiology:

Ehlers-Danlos Syndrome is generally autosomal dominant, but up to 50% may occur from de novo mutations. Each subtype correlates with specific genetic mutations affecting various collagen types and other extracellular matrix proteins.

Hypermobility Spectrum Disorders:

HSDs are conditions related to EDS, particularly the hypermobile subtype. These disorders are characterized by generalized joint hypermobility but do not fulfill the criteria for any of the EDS subtypes. Although they share some features, they are considered separate from EDS and do not have known genetic markers.

In individuals with EDS and HSD, the connective tissue that helps maintain the body's structural integrity is weaker than normal. This also affects the ligaments and soft tissues supporting the cervical spine, making them more lax and prone to instability. The cervical spine bears the weight of the head and allows for its diverse range of motion. Instability in this area can lead to a variety of neurological symptoms and complications. It may be due to shifting vertebral segments or a form of muscle guarding that leads to compressive forces placed on the carotid sheath where the vagus nerve lies. This can result in vagus nerve dysfunction due to either transient or constant compression. Patients may then present with high or low vagal tone symptoms or a mixture.

References

1. Bascom, R., Dhingra, R. and Francomano, C.A., 2021. Respiratory manifestations in the Ehlers-Danlos syndromes. Am J Med Genet C Semin Med Genet, 187(4), pp.533-548.

2. Borg, I., Formosa, M.M., Farrugia, R. and Scicluna, K., 2022. hypermobile Ehlers-Danlos syndrome: A review and a critical appraisal of published genetic research to date. Clin Genet, 101(1), pp.20-31.

3. Borge, R., Kamps-Schmitt, K.A. and Yew, K.S., 2021. Hypermobile Ehlers-Danlos Syndrome and Hypermobility Spectrum Disorders. Am Fam Physician, 103(8), pp.481-492.

4. Burgell, R.E., Gibson, P.R. and Thwaites, P.A., 2022. Hypermobile Ehlers-Danlos syndrome and disorders of the gastrointestinal tract: What the gastroenterologist needs to know. J Gastroenterol hepatol, 37(9), pp.1693-1709.

5. Caty, G., De Backer, M.M., Piraux, E., Poncin, W. and Reychler, G., 2021. Physical therapy treatment of hypermobile Ehlers-Danlos syndrome: A systematic review. Am J Med Genet A, 185(10), pp.2986-2994.

6. Davidar, A.D., Hersh, A.M., Jin, Y., Kopparapu, S., Mao, G., Theodore, N. and Weber-Levine, C., 2022. Craniocervical instability in patients with Ehlers-Danlos syndrome: controversies in diagnosis and management. Spine J, 22(12), pp.1944-1952.

7. Gensemer, C., Burks, R., Judge, D.P., Kautz, S., Lavallee, M. and Norris, R.A., 2021. hypermobile Ehlers-Danlos syndromes: Complex phenotypes, challenging diagnoses, and poorly understood causes. Dev Dyn, 250(3), pp.318-344.

8. Guerrieri, V., Polizzi, A., Caliogna, L., Brancato, A.M., Bassotti, A., Torriani, C., Jannelli, E., Mosconi, M., Grassi, F.A. and Pasta, G., 2023. Pain in Ehlers-Danlos Syndrome: A Non-Diagnostic Disabling Symptom? healthcare (Basel), 11(7), p.936.

9. Hakim, A., Iodice, V., Mathias, C.J. and Owens, A., 2021. Dysautonomia in the Ehlers-Danlos syndromes and hypermobility spectrum disorders-With a focus on the postural tachycardia syndrome. Am J Med Genet C Semin Med Genet, 187(4), pp.510-519.

10. Han, S.J. and Royer, S.P., 2022. Mechanobiology in the Comorbidities of Ehlers-Danlos Syndrome. Front Cell Dev Biol, 10, p.874840.

11. Lam, C.M., Wood, G. and Birchall, M.A., 2022. Laryngological presentations and patient-reported outcome measures in Ehlers-Danlos syndrome. J Laryngol Otol, 136(10), pp.947-951.

12. Miklovic, T. and Sieg, V.C., 2023. Ehlers-Danlos Syndrome. In: StatPearls. Treasure Island (FL): StatPearls Publishing

Chapter 35
Mast Cell Activation Syndrome

Mast cells are specialized cells of the immune system involved in allergy responses and inflammation. They are found in various tissues throughout the body, including the skin, lungs, and digestive system. In Mast Cell Activation Syndrome, these cells are hyper-responsive, leading to excessive degranulation and release of various chemicals and mediators, such as histamine. Understanding MCAS is crucial because of its multi-system involvement and the significant impact it can have on an individual's quality of life.

The signs and symptoms of Mast Cell Activation Syndrome (MCAS) are incredibly diverse, reflecting the widespread distribution of mast cells throughout the body. Patients may experience a myriad of symptoms that can differ significantly from one individual to another. Dermatological symptoms may include hives, itching, angioedema, flushing, and dermatographia, while respiratory issues might manifest as wheezing, shortness of breath, or cough. The gastrointestinal tract can also be affected, leading to abdominal pain, nausea, vomiting, and diarrhea. Neurologically, patients may report migraines, brain fog, and fatigue. On the cardiovascular front, symptoms can range from palpitations and low blood pressure to tachycardia. Additionally, some patients experience other symptoms such as bone or muscle pain, anaphylaxis, and sensitivity to temperature changes, scents, and chemicals, along with anxiety or mood swings.

These diverse manifestations make the diagnosis and management of MCAS a complex endeavor, requiring a multi-systemic approach to accurately identify and treat the condition. The variability of symptoms not only makes it challenging for healthcare providers to pin down a diagnosis but also impacts the quality of life for those suffering from this perplexing syndrome.

The etiology of Mast Cell Activation Syndrome (MCAS) is complex and not fully understood, encompassing a range of suspected contributing factors. Familial patterns have led researchers to consider genetic factors as a potential influence, although no specific genes have been conclusively identified. Environmental factors, such as exposure to toxins or allergens, are also thought to predispose individuals to MCAS. Additionally, viral and bacterial infections have been suspected as potential triggers that could lead to mast cell activation. The role of autoimmunity in MCAS is still a subject of ongoing research but is increasingly considered a plausible contributory factor. Despite these avenues of investigation, a significant number of cases remain idiopathic, with no identifiable cause, underscoring the multifactorial and elusive nature of this syndrome.

Diagnosing Mast Cell Activation Syndrome (MCAS) is a complex task, made especially challenging by its myriad symptoms that can affect multiple organ systems and the absence of a single, definitive diagnostic test. Clinicians often rely on a combination of criteria to arrive at a diagnosis. The clinical criteria require the presence of symptoms impacting at least two organ systems, which could range from dermatological to gastrointestinal to neurological issues. Laboratory criteria involve the detection of elevated levels of mast cell mediators, such as tryptase, histamine, or prostaglandin D2, ideally measured during a symptomatic episode to capture the most accurate reflection of mast cell activity. Finally, the response to treatment is also considered a supportive pillar for diagnosis; an improvement in symptoms upon the administration of medications like antihistamines or mast cell stabilizers often strengthens the case for an MCAS diagnosis. This multi-pronged approach is designed to capture the wide variability in symptoms and experiences, aiming to offer a comprehensive diagnostic framework for this elusive syndrome.

To diagnose Mast Cell Activation Syndrome (MCAS), a variety of tests are often utilized, each with its own set of advantages and limitations. The Serum Tryptase test, which measures the level of tryptase in the blood, is the most commonly used marker. However, it's crucial to note that levels may not always be elevated even during symptomatic episodes, making it an imperfect diagnostic tool. The 24-hour Urine Test for N-methylhistamine aims to measure histamine metabolites excreted in the urine over a day and can sometimes be more sensitive than serum histamine levels for detecting mast cell activation. Prostaglandin D2 levels can also be assessed; elevated levels may indicate mast cell activation but are not specific to MCAS, thereby requiring further tests for conclusive diagnosis. In more ambiguous cases, a Bone Marrow Biopsy may be conducted. Though invasive, this test can help rule out mastocytosis, a condition that shares many symptoms with MCAS. These multiple testing approaches reflect the complexity of diagnosing MCAS and the need for a comprehensive evaluation to capture its varying presentations.

Other conditions with similar presentations need to be ruled out, such as:

- Hereditary Alpha-tryptasemia Syndrome
- Systemic Mastocytosis
- Idiopathic Anaphylaxis
- Various autoimmune and gastrointestinal disorders

The Vagus Nerve and Mast Cell Activation Syndrome:

The vagus nerve plays a significant role in the regulation of inflammatory responses through the cholinergic anti-inflammatory pathway. Activation of the vagus nerve has been shown to inhibit pro-inflammatory cytokine release and reduce inflammation in various experimental models. Dysfunction of the vagus nerve could disrupt this regulatory pathway, contributing to uncontrolled inflammation and subsequent mast cell activation.

Dysregulation of Neurotransmitters and Hormones:

The vagus nerve is instrumental in the release and regulation of neurotransmitters like acetylcholine and hormones like cortisol.

Dysfunctional vagus nerve activity may lead to imbalances in these neurochemicals, potentially triggering mast cell degranulation, thereby leading to symptoms of MCAS.

Gut-Brain Axis Disruption:

The vagus nerve plays a critical role in maintaining the gut-brain axis. Vagal dysfunction may disrupt gut motility and barrier function, leading to increased intestinal permeability. Such "leaky gut" could then lead to the translocation of bacteria and their products, such as lipopolysaccharides, which can activate mast cells.

Direct Mast Cell-Vagus Nerve Interaction:

Recent research has begun to elucidate the direct interactions between the vagus nerve and mast cells. Some mast cells reside in close proximity to vagal nerve fibers, and there is evidence that mast cells can be directly activated or inhibited by signals from the vagus nerve. Thus, dysfunctional vagal signaling could directly contribute to inappropriate mast cell activation.

While the relationship between vagus nerve dysfunction and MCAS is still being actively researched, existing evidence suggests multiple pathways through which vagal dysfunction could contribute to mast cell activation. Understanding this relationship more fully will require further study but has the potential to open new avenues for the treatment and management of MCAS.

References

1. Afrin, L. B., Self, S., Menk, J., & Lazarchick, J. (2017). Characterization of Mast Cell Activation Syndrome. The American Journal of the Medical Sciences, 353(3), 207-215.

2. Akin, C., Valent, P., & Metcalfe, D. D. (2010). Mast cell activation syndrome: Proposed diagnostic criteria. Journal of Allergy and Clinical Immunology, 126(6), 1099-1104.

3. Bonaz, B., Sinniger, V., & Pellissier, S. (2017). The Vagus Nerve in the Neuro-Immune Axis: Implications in the Pathology of the Gastrointestinal Tract. Frontiers in Immunology, 8, 1452.

4. Hamilton, M. J., Hornick, J. L., Akin, C., Castells, M. C., & Greenberger, N. J. (2011). Mast cell activation syndrome: A newly recognized disorder with systemic clinical manifestations. Journal of Allergy and Clinical Immunology, 128(1), 147-152.

5. Tracey, K. J. (2007). Physiology and immunology of the cholinergic anti-inflammatory pathway. The Journal of Clinical Investigation, 117(2), 289-296.

6. Valent, P., Akin, C., Bonadonna, P., Hartmann, K., & Brockow, K. (2021). Why the 20% + 2 Tryptase Formula Is a Diagnostic Gold Standard for Severe Systemic Mast Cell Activation and Mast Cell Activation Syndrome. International Archives of Allergy and Immunology, 182(4), 265-278.

Chapter 36
Is It All One disease?

The vast array of symptoms that individuals present — from mood fluctuations and alterations in voice to irregular heart rates, digestive complications, respiratory issues, and the pervasive brain fog — leaves both medical professionals and patients in a state of perplexity. The myriad of conditions that these symptoms indicate seem distinct, almost unrelated at first glance. Yet, could there be a singular thread weaving them together? Emerging research is pointing towards vagus nerve dysfunction as the potential common denominator. In this culminating chapter, we aim to traverse the intricate landscape of these symptoms, shed light on the possible nexus through vagus nerve dysfunction — frequently rooted in cervical instability — and delve into therapeutic approaches, including nerve manipulation, cervical strengthening, and transcutaneous auricular vagus nerve stimulation (taVNS), which could present a comprehensive remedy.

The Vagus Nerve: Unraveling the Mystery

While the vagus nerve has often been overshadowed in common medical discussions, its critical role in the human body is undeniable. Not only does it act as a communication superhighway between the brain and multiple organs, but its influence permeates a variety of physiological functions. It's becoming increasingly clear that disturbances in this nerve can ripple across the body, leading to a cascade of symptoms that, on the surface, appear unrelated.

Mood alterations, for example, aren't just products of the brain alone. They can be influenced by the gut, often termed the 'second brain', which relies on the vagus nerve for communication. Voice changes might hint at laryngeal muscle dysfunction, another domain of the vagus nerve. The rhythm of our heart, the movement of food through our gut, our very breath — all fall under the purview of this extensive nerve. Hence, a disruption in its function can be like throwing a wrench into the cogs of a machine, affecting its entire operation.

Cervical Instability: A Potential Keystone

One might wonder, what could be causing this widespread vagus nerve dysfunction? Enter cervical instability. The cervical spine, tasked with the crucial job of supporting the head and safeguarding the neural pathways, plays an even more pivotal role when it comes to the vagus nerve. Instability or misalignment here can lead to compression or irritation of the nerve, setting off a chain reaction of symptoms throughout the body. Recognizing this connection might be the key to unlocking the mystery behind the array of symptoms that have baffled so many for so long.

Towards a Holistic Therapeutic Future

With this newfound understanding, the direction for treatment becomes clear: address the root. Nerve manipulation techniques, specifically designed to free entrapped nerves, can restore their natural function. Strengthening exercises targeting the cervical region can alleviate instability, offering the nerve a more protective, stable environment. Additionally, innovations like taVNS bring forth non-invasive ways to enhance the vagus nerve's function directly, showing promise in symptom relief across the board.

In Conclusion: A Paradigm Shift in Understanding

As we stand on the cusp of this medical revelation, the paradigm of understanding diverse symptoms and conditions is shifting. No longer might we need to treat each symptom in isolation. Instead, by focusing on the underlying commonality — the vagus nerve — and its relationship with cervical stability, we could usher in an era of holistic, integrated healthcare. This journey of discovery holds not just the promise of more effective treatments but also the hope of transforming countless lives by treating the root, not just the branches.

Epilogue:
The Harmonious Symphony of the Vagus Nerve

In the winding pathways of our body, a quiet luminary exists – the vagus nerve. Through our exploration of its intricate anatomy and multifaceted physiology, we've unearthed the significant role this cranial nerve plays in the grand orchestration of human health.

Its tendrils, reaching deep into our very core, modulate our heart rate, assist in digesting the foods that sustain us, and carry the whispers of our organs back to the awaiting ears of the brain. Our bodies, in many ways, hinge on the seamless operations commanded by the vagus nerve.

Yet, as we delved into its potential therapeutic applications, the vagus nerve's true brilliance emerged. Vagus Nerve Stimulation (VNS) has opened doors to new treatments for conditions previously deemed challenging, forging pathways of hope for many.

Beyond what we've discovered about its immediate implications in health and disease, the vagus nerve stands as a testament to the interconnectedness of our body systems. It challenges the compartmentalized approach often taken in medicine, urging us to consider the body as a holistic entity where changes in one area resonate throughout.

As we stand on the precipice of future research and clinical applications, it's clear that our journey with the vagus nerve is far from over. Every new discovery not only propels the medical community forward but also deepens our respect for this intricate neural highway. The coming years will undoubtedly bring forth innovations, refining our understanding and harnessing the vagus nerve's potential even further.

THE VAGUS NERVE

To the students, educators, and practitioners who have journeyed through this book, may you carry forth the knowledge with both humility and enthusiasm. Let the vagus nerve serve as a reminder that within the minutiae of our bodily systems lies a vast, harmonious symphony waiting to be understood.

In the quest for knowledge and in service to humanity, may we always be guided by curiosity, empathy, and the profound interconnectedness of all life.

Glossary of Terms:

A

- Acetylcholine: A neurotransmitter used by neurons in both the sympathetic and parasympathetic nervous systems.
- Adrenergic: Refers to nerve cells in which adrenaline, noradrenaline, or similar substances act as neurotransmitters.
- Afferent Neurons: Neurons that carry sensory information from the body to the central nervous system.
- Autonomic Ganglia: Clusters of nerve cell bodies in the ANS.

B

- Baroreceptors: Pressure-sensitive sensory neurons that respond to changes in blood pressure.
- Brainstem: The part of the brain that connects the cerebrum with the spinal cord and houses the origins of the vagus nerve.

C

- Cardioinhibitory Center: Part of the medulla oblongata that receives inputs from baroreceptors and modulates heart rate via the vagus nerve.
- Celiac Ganglion: A large ganglion in the ANS that receives fibers from the splanchnic nerves and sends fibers to the abdominal viscera.
- Central Nervous System (CNS): The part of the nervous system consisting of the brain and spinal cord.

THE HARMONIOUS SYMPHONY OF THE VAGUS NERVE

D
- Dorsal Motor Nucleus: A group of neurons in the medulla oblongata that provides parasympathetic innervation to the heart via the vagus nerve.

E
- Efferent Neurons: Neurons that carry motor commands from the central nervous system to muscles and glands.
- Enteric Nervous System: A subdivision of the ANS controlling the gastrointestinal system, with connections to the vagus nerve.

F
- Fight-or-Flight Response: A physiological reaction mediated by the sympathetic nervous system in response to stress or perceived threat.

G
- Ganglion: A cluster of nerve cell bodies located outside the CNS.

H
- Homeostasis: The ability of an organism to maintain internal equilibrium by adjusting its physiological processes.

I
- Interoception: The sense of the internal state of the body, facilitated in part by the vagus nerve.

M
- Medulla Oblongata: The lower part of the brainstem, containing control centers for the heart and lungs, including vagus nerve nuclei.

N
- Neurotransmitter: A chemical messenger that transmits signals across a nerve synapse.
- Norepinephrine: A neurotransmitter and hormone important in the fight-or-flight response.

P

- Parasympathetic Nervous System: One of the two main divisions of the ANS, often called the "rest and digest" system.
- Peripheral Nervous System (PNS): The nervous system outside the brain and spinal cord, including the ANS.
- Preganglionic Neuron: The first neuron in a series that transmits impulses from the CNS to an autonomic ganglion.

S

- Sympathetic Nervous System: One of the two main divisions of the ANS, often called the "fight or flight" system.
- Sympathetic Chain: A chain of ganglia that runs down each side of the spinal column, part of the sympathetic division of the ANS.
- Synapse: The junction between two nerve cells, consisting of a minuscule gap across which impulses pass by diffusion of a neurotransmitter.

T

- Thoracic Outflow: The sympathetic nerves emerging from the thoracic spinal cord that innervate organs above the diaphragm.
- Tonic Activity: Continuous or baseline activity of neurons.

V

- Vagotomy: Surgical cutting of the vagus nerve to reduce acid secretion in the stomach.
- Vagus Nerve: The tenth cranial nerve, part of the parasympathetic system, which influences heart rate, digestion, and other functions.
- Vagal Tone: The activity of the vagus nerve, influencing heart rate variability and reflecting the balance of the autonomic nervous system.
- Visceral Reflexes: Involuntary reflexes controlled by the autonomic nervous system to regulate the function of internal organs.

About The Author

Emrys Goldsworthy's journey through life is a tapestry of art and science. With an illustrious career as a professional ballet dancer with the Royal New Zealand Ballet, Emrys gracefully transitioned his understanding of human anatomy from the dance studio to the clinic. Boasting over 15 years as a Musculoskeletal Therapist, his expertise in the human body is both profound and multifaceted.

A beacon of knowledge, Emrys served as a senior lecturer at the Endeavour College of Natural Health for close to a decade. His thirst for innovation and deep understanding of therapeutic techniques led him to design and teach pioneering courses on nerve manipulation, shockwave therapy, and dry needling for more than 13 years.

Though his roots in ballet never waned, Emrys continued to contribute to the art, choreographing pieces and, more recently, taking the helm as the Artistic Director of Ballet Infinity.

Today, Emrys resides in Australia, where he seamlessly marries his dual passions for health and ballet, showcasing the symbiotic relationship between discipline, art, and the intricate wonders of the human body.

For more information on Emrys Goldsworthy's clinic and educational programs go to **www.emrysgoldsworthy.com.au**

Printed in Great Britain
by Amazon